Seventh-day Adventist Health Reform—
A Crucible of Identity Tensions

Seventh-day Adventist Health Reform—A Crucible of Identity Tensions

Ellen G. White and Dr. John H. Kellogg—
The Battle for Seventh-day Adventist Identity

RICHARD B. FERRET

PICKWICK *Publications* · Eugene, Oregon

SEVENTH-DAY ADVENTIST HEALTH REFORM—A CRUCIBLE
OF IDENTITY TENSIONS
Ellen G. White and Dr. John H. Kellogg—The Battle for Seventh-day
Adventist Identity

Pickwick Publications
An Imprint of Wipf and Stock Publishers
199 W. 8th Ave., Suite 3
Eugene, OR 97401

www.wipfandstock.com

PAPERBACK ISBN: 978-1-6667-7455-9
HARDCOVER ISBN: 978-1-6667-7456-6
EBOOK ISBN: 978-1-6667-7457-3

Cataloguing-in-Publication data:

Names: Ferret, Richard B. (Richard Bowen), author.

Title: Seventh-day Adventist health reform—a crucible of identity tensions : Ellen G. White and Dr. John H. Kellogg—The Battle for Seventh-day Adventist Identity / Richard B. Ferret.

Description: Eugene, OR: Pickwick Publications, 2023. | Includes bibliographical references.

Identifiers: ISBN 978-1-6667-7455-9 (paperback). | ISBN 978-1-6667-7456-6 (hardcover). | ISBN 978-1-6667-7457-3 (ebook).

Subjects: LSCH: Seventh-day Adventists—History. | White, Ellen G., 1827–1915. | Kellogg, John H., 1852–1943. | Health care.

Classification: BX6193.W5 F45 2023 (print). | BX6193 (ebook).

07/07/23

Copyright Permission granted by Herbert Richardson, Editor for the Edwin Mellen Press.

I dedicate this book to my wife, Jenny, and our three children,
Anthony, Beau & Ashlee

Contents

1

Introduction

IN 1893 THE SEVENTH-DAY Adventist Medical Missionary and Benevolent Association was established by the General Conference of the Seventh-day Adventist (SDA) church in Battle Creek, Michigan under the leadership of Dr. John Harvey Kellogg, MD, who, apart from Ellen G. White influenced the philosophy and global development of SDA health reform more than any other individual. Historically, John Harvey Kellogg was undoubtedly the most-well known and recognized Seventh-day Adventist of that era. His small stature, but 'larger than life' persona have been well documented, and the Kellogg name is still emblazoned across breakfast cereals, which are consumed on a daily basis around the world. He was one of America's early biostatisticians and influential preventative health practitioners who sought to provide, among many things, scientific evidence to undergird White's counsels on health reform (Schwarz, 2006: 9). Indeed, Kellogg was one of the few Adventists of his time to take White's views on health reform seriously (Bull & Lockhart, 2007: 302).

By 1896, the medical leaders at Battle Creek voted successfully for a name change of the organization that substituted 'Seventh-day Adventist' to 'International.' The rationale for this change of nomenclature was designed to reflect the increasingly global scope of Adventist growth. However, another reason for the name change was provided in the January 1898 issue of *Medical Missionary* by Dr. Kellogg:

The International Medical Missionary and Benevolent Association is a unique organization in the fact that it is, as far as we know at least, the only association which has undertaken to organize and carry forward medical and philanthropic work *independent of any sectarian or denominational control,* in home and foreign lands (emphasis mine).

Tensions soon became patently evident between church administrators, ministers, White, and Kellogg and his associates concerning the word 'denominational' when applied to the function and operation of the Association. The agents of the Medical Missionary and Benevolent Association insisted that their existence centered on being "here as Christians, and not as Seventh-day Adventists." In a similar vein in 1899, at a convention of the Association, the delegates declared that their purpose was not to present anything "that is peculiarly Seventh-day Adventist in doctrine," rather, their work was "simply the undenominational side of the work which Seventh-day Adventists have to do in the world" (Kellogg, 1899).

For many Adventists the growing number of declarations such as these by Dr. Kellogg and his connections provided serious cause for alarm. Previously in 1893, Kellogg had authored an article titled "Fraternity in Missionary Work," in which he made a plea for recruits to become properly trained medical missionaries, including both physicians and nurses. In addition, he made the following observations, the implications of which are clearly discernable:

A hundred could be set to work at once in this country alone. Such missionaries are wanted, not to engage in proselytizing men and women to a creed, not for the purpose of disseminating a doctrine or doctrines, but to help lift fallen men and women to a higher moral level through the alleviation of their physical sufferings and the amelioration of their physical wants and necessities . . . If Christians would only tear themselves away from the narrowness of self and the bigotry of church pride and denominationalism, and devote themselves to earnest work for their fellow men . . . the gibes of the infidel and the scorner would soon be silenced (Medical Missionary, March-April, 1893).

Two years later when announcing the opening of the American Medical Missionary College, Kellogg was again emphatic in his declaration:

This is not a sectarian school. Sectarian doctrines are not to be taught in this medical school. It is a school for the purpose of teaching medical science, theoretically and practically, and gospel missionary work. It is not to be either a Seventh-day Adventist or a Methodist or a Baptist, or any other sectarian school, but a Christian medical college, to which all Christian men and Christian women who are ready to devote their lives to Christian work will be admitted (Medical Missionary, October, 1895).

White vehemently opposed both Kellogg's, and the Association's view that the American Medical Missionary College was being announced to the world as providing an 'undenominational' charter. Shortly after the opening of the medical school White wrote a letter to the medical superintendent of the sanitarium emphasizing, in no uncertain terms, that "the remnant people of God" were to glorify God's name by "proclaiming the last message of warning," and the *only* method in which God's remnant Adventists could achieve this goal was "by being representatives of the truth for this time" (8T: 153). While in the same letter White commended Kellogg for having once "stood nobly for the faith once delivered to the saints," she insisted that he now faced his sternest test. Kellogg's dangerous position was symbolically described by White:

> I saw you holding up the banner on which are written the words, 'Here is the patience of the saints; here are they that keep the commandments of God, and the faith of Jesus.' Revelation 14:12. Several men, some of them those with whom you are connected in the sanitarium, were presenting to you a banner which was a different inscription. You were letting go the banner of Seventh-day Adventists. . . . I was instructed that you and your fellow laborers were in danger of hiding the principles of the faith in order to obtain large patronage. Every jot done in this line, instead of extending the influence of truth, will hinder its advance (8T: 153, 154).

White provided further admonition insisting that no concealing of the distinctive truths of Adventism would be countenanced, accept at a severe cost. In addition, she declared that there would be no covering up of any phase of our message, and no narrowing down of the Doctor's work. "The truth for this time," she stated, "must be given to the souls ready to perish. Those who in any way hide the truth dishonor God. Upon their garments will be the blood of souls" (8T: 155). Concerning the identity of the Battle Creek Sanitarium, White continued in unequivocal terms:

> It has been stated that the Battle Creek Sanitarium is not denominational. But if ever an institution was established to be

denominational, in every sense of the word, this sanitarium was. Why are sanitariums established if it is not that they may be the right hand of the gospel in calling the attention of men and women to the truth that we are living amid the perils of the last days? Any yet, in one sense, it is true that the Battle Creek Sanitarium is undenominational, in that it receives as patients people of all classes and denominations (5 Bio: 160).

Finally, the co-founder of Seventh-day Adventism made her position concerning SDA institutional identity decidedly unambiguous:

> Now and ever we are to stand as a distinct and peculiar people, free from all worldly policy, unembarrassed by confederating with those who have not wisdom to discern the claims of God, so plainly set forth in His law. We are not to take pains to declare that the Battle Creek Sanitarium is not a Seventh-day Adventist institution, for it certainly is. As a Seventh—day Adventist institution, it was established, to represent the various features of gospel missionary work, thus to prepare the way for the coming of the Lord (5Bio: 160).

By 1906 the escalation of tensions between key leaders of Adventism's medical work who were located primarily in Battle Creek under the direction of Dr. Kellogg and the church leaders, who were primarily from a ministerial background had escalated to the point of irreparable rupture and separation. Such was the struggle that the burgeoning question at the commencement of the twentieth century in Adventism was whether the movement would remain clerically dominated or follow Kellogg's mandate for his medicalized version of Seventh-day Adventism, which was fundamentally different from the church leadership and mainstream membership. In essence, Kellogg advocated a social gospel devoid of sectarian constraints, arguing that being a 'Good Samaritan' in society was more important than being a good theologian or minister, and that humanitarian work would prove more successful for the Adventist cause then all the church's clergy efforts combined.

Bull and Lockhart argue forcefully that Dr. Kellogg could approach society as a medical professional, with a mission to heal, rather than damn other Americans as the Adventist clergy were well noted for, and this was a significant factor in his revulsion of Adventist sectarianism. Ultimately, Kellogg set the medical work at odds with both the church administrators and ministry declaring the medical work "independent of denominational control" (2007: 304). White's rebuke of Kellogg consisted of more than a clarification of minor differences or definitions; it was an attempt to jettison his "redefining the nature of Adventism," including a "diminution of Adventist distinctiveness" that by the 1890s threatened to alter Adventism's identity in relationship to the American republic (Bull & Lockhart, 2007: 302, 303).

In 1904, in the midst of a theological crisis in Adventism (pantheism), White anticipating the ensuing breach in Adventism, delivered an address to delegates at a Union Conference session in Berrien Springs, calling for unity between ministers and medical trained personnel:

> My brethren, the Lord calls for unity, for oneness. We are to be of one faith. I want to tell you that when the gospel ministers and the medical missionaries workers are not united, there is placed in our churches the worst evil that can be placed there. Our medical missionaries ought to be interested in the work of our conferences, and our conference workers ought to be as much interested in the work of our medical missionaries (MM: 241).

Of immense significance is that while both White and Kellogg spoke of the *gospel medical missionary work* as being essential in benefiting humankind, their interpretation and understanding of that same work was fundamentally different. In other words, the future direction of SDA health care and institutions was at stake. In effect, the basis of Kellogg's 'biological living' health reform endeavors placed his medical world on a divergent path from White's and traditional Adventism, thus impacting the movement's ongoing identity. The sanitarium he created interfaced with society on humanitarian and medical grounds rather than on a specifically Adventist foundation that was clerically dominated.

For Kellogg, the key to salvation consisted of making people well and maintaining that condition. Wilson argues that the core essence of Kellogg's emphasis concerned biological living (2014). Thus, one's state of health, and not one's theology was Kellogg's mandate (Bull & Lockhart, 2007: 303). White, conversely, considered health reform an important element in the salvation process, but it was secondary to the theological foundations of the Seventh-day Adventist message of warning to an increasingly degenerate and dying world. White systematically referred to the health message as the 'right arm' of the body (6T: 327). Her sense of eschatological urgency is apparent in her unequivocal assessment of the balance required between the 'arm' and the 'body'

The health reform is as closely related to the third angel's message as the arm to the body; but the arm cannot take the place of the body. The proclamation of the third angel's message, the commandments of God, and the testimony of Jesus is the great burden of our work. The message is to be proclaimed with a loud cry, and is to go to the whole world. The presentation of health principles must be united with this message, but must not in any case be independent of it, or in any way take the place of it (CW: 139).

The irreconcilable differences between White and Kellogg regarding the nature and function of the medical ministry work was not limited to the control of SDA medical institutions, and the ensuing separation between the ministry and medical professions in institutionalized Adventism. Rather, the nature of Adventist identity in the world was at stake. The question as to which model of institutionalized health care (White's or Kellogg's) exists today provides a rationale for this research.

Prior to considering nineteenth century American health reform it is important to briefly consider the impact of institutionalization on Seventh-day Adventism, for this evaluation provides a broader context in which to assess the different trajectories between White and Kellogg regarding the nature of their respective medical models.

Seventh-day Adventist Institutionalization and Identity

If you approached a Seventh-day Adventist from any region of the world in 2023 and enquired as to what constitutes or defines their religious identity, it would be highly likely that the majority would frame their response in relation to their theological beliefs. For example, "I believe in the seventh-day Sabbath and the soon coming, literal return of Jesus Christ to earth," both teachings which are inherent in the name Seventh-day Adventist. It would be of interest if any Adventists would respond by declaring that their church is a wealthy, constantly developing, multi-national movement with significant organizational and institutional (educational, medical, publishing, health foods etc.) structures that appear to be succeeding quite well in today's societies, yet nonetheless, would appear very foreign to their pioneers.

It is estimated that by the year 2050 more than 6 out of 10 people on planet Earth will be either Muslim or Christian, and, for perhaps the first time in history, Islam and Christianity could boast roughly equal numbers equating to almost 3 billion adherents each. Within the Protestant Christian tradition, Seventh-day Adventism is one of the fastest growing churches in the world today, experiencing a growth rate of 7% in some regions in the 3rd decade of the 21st century. In 2013, G. T. Ng, executive secretary of the SDA world church, told church leaders during his report at the Annual Council in Silver Spring, Maryland, United States that "on any given day 3,052 people join the church. Every hour 127 people are baptized. Every minute, two individuals are baptized, and we praise God for that."

Seventh-day Adventism emerged as a premillennial, eschatologically focused movement during the Second Great Awakening in mid-nineteenth century North America, with Ellen G. White as its dominant prophetic figure. Other charismatic leaders were also instrumental during the same historical period in producing such enduring traditions as the Christian Scientists, Latter Day Saints, and Jehovah's Witnesses, along with the emergence of Spiritualism. This period in American history, also known as the Jacksonian era, was renowned for its political, social, scientific, cultural and religious upheavals, during which the country was swamped with innovation and change impacting almost all facets of life. These stressful and confusing, yet exciting times, provided an opportune climate for millennial movements to materialize and flourish by providing new assumptions, new redemptive processes, new political and economic boundaries, new communities and new models for measuring humanity and in many cases, a new "prophet" to organize and articulate these new assumptions (Butler, 1993: 189).

The SDA church defines itself as a prophetic remnant, raised up and commissioned by God to preach a unique and final message of warning to the world, prior to the visible and climactic return of the Lord Jesus Christ to earth, as portrayed particularly in the biblical books of Daniel and Revelation as well as throughout the New Testament.

Ellen White (1827–1915), cofounder of the SDA movement, declared the cultural attitudes of the movement:

> Every institution that bears the name of Seventh-day Adventist is to be to the world as was Joseph in Egypt, and as were Daniel and his fellows in Babylon. In the providence of God these men were taken captive, that they might carry to heathen nations the knowledge of the true God. They were to make no compromise with the idolatrous nations with which they were brought in contact, but were to stand loyal to their faith, bearing as a special

honor the name of worshippers of the God who created the heavens and the earth (8T: 153).

God designed that the institutions [sanitariums] which He should establish should stand forth as a beacon of light, of warning and reproof. He would prove to the world that an institution conducted on religious principles, as an asylum for the sick, could be sustained without sacrificing its peculiar, holy character; that it could be kept free from the objectionable features found in other health institutions. It was to be an instrument for bringing about great reforms (6T: 223).

Growth produced its own problems, however:

As our work has extended and institutions have multiplied, God's purpose in their establishment remains the same. The conditions of prosperity are unchanged (6T: 224).

Towards the end of the twentieth century, the drift in this last statement of denial was apparent to scholars, and indicative of the identity dilemmas confronting the movement:

There is a definite sense in which failure was built into the very success of the young denomination. That is, in order to preserve the message of the imminent coming [of Christ], institutions based on continuity and semi-permanence had to be erected. And in the process subtle and not–so–subtle transformations took place (Knight, 1995: 153).

The global SDA church in the 3rd decade of the twenty-first century is very different from the fledgling movement formally organized in North America in 1863. While statistics provide only a limited perspective, they do offer an insight into an ever-increasing SDA membership that has grown from a few thousand in the 1860s to over 20 million members in 2020, with current predictions estimating that church membership worldwide could reach 30 million by 2030. The ratio of church members to world population in 1863 was 1: 373,143; early in 2014 it stood at 1: 403. As of September 30, 2020 there were 20,802 active ordained ministers and 323,072 other employees working for the SDA church with over 91,000 organized churches and a further 72, 605 companies in existence.

Of the 275 countries and regions of the world recognized by the United Nations, SDA's have an established presence in 215. The Adventist educational system boasts 9,489 schools globally with a total enrollment of over 2 million students. Health care facilities include 227 hospitals and sanitariums, 133 nursing home and retirement centers, 673 clinics and dispensaries, 15 orphanages and children's homes with outpatient visits to the various health services totaling over 20 million. 60 publishing houses and branches operate worldwide and publish in 311 languages, while 23 food industries operate. ADRA (Adventist Development and Relief Agency International) functions in over 118 countries, and the beneficiaries of ADRA projects was 13,940,983. Monetary support of the church through personal tithes and offerings in 2018 was almost US$3 billion.

The GDP register by both the United Nations and World Bank lists 193 countries on its database with the United States ranked first and Tuvalu, a small Polynesian island nation located in the Pacific Ocean ranked last. If the SDA church were deemed a nation, it would rank 159/193 in relation to income through tithes and offerings alone, placing the church's financial income above nations such as the Solomon Islands, Tonga, Samoa, Liberia, Andorra, Burundi, Greenland etc. When Adventism's pioneering prophet Ellen White died in 1915, the assets of the movement were estimated to be less than US$12 million; in 2020 (recognizing inflation) conservative estimates totaled over US$20 billion, excluding churches and primary schools.

Based on this statistical information, one might assume that the SDA church would be well known and recognized globally. Bull and Lockhart, in arguably the most insightful and provocative analysis of Seventh-day Adventism to date, argue otherwise. In their book, *Seeking a Sanctuary: Seventh-day Adventism and the American Dream* the authors cite a survey conducted in North America in 2003 in which 44% of the respondents declared that they had never heard of Seventh-day Adventism. Of those who had heard of Adventism, approximately two thirds were able to provide some further information. Some were aware that the SDA church was "a religion," while many knew that Saturday was observed as the Sabbath day of worship. 15% confused Adventists with either Jehovah's Witnesses or the Mormons. Apart from the Saturday Sabbath, awareness of the church's practices and beliefs were vague. One in fifteen knew of an Adventist hospital in their vicinity, but among those who confused Adventists and Jehovah's Witnesses, the SDA church was believed to resist blood transfusions. Altogether, a third of respondents viewed Adventism positively, while a fifth perceived it negatively (2007: 1). The same authors contend that Seventh-day Adventism is "one of the most subtly differentiated, systematically developed, and institutionally successful of all alternatives to the American way of life:

> A nineteenth-century religious sect that observes a seventh-day Sabbath, proclaims the imminent end of the world, and practices health reform, Seventh-day Adventism is now on the way to becoming a major religion. . . . During the last century, it consistently doubled its membership every fifteen years or less, with the rate accelerating over time. . . . Although its membership has overtaken that of the Latter-day Saints and the Jehovah Witnesses, Seventh-day Adventism is still largely ignored (2007: xiii).

Joshua Himes, a faithful supporter of William Miller, wrote to Ellen White in 1895, a half-century after the Millerite Great Disappointment of 1844, highlighting, as he saw it, the dilemma facing the movement:

> You have many good and great things connected with health reform and the churches, with the increase in wealth, and colleges as well, and to me it looks like work in all these departments that may go on for a long time to come. . . . There is a great and earnest work being done to send the message of the third angel everywhere-but all classes of Adventists are prospering in worldly things, and heaping up riches, while they talk of the coming of Christ as an event very near at hand. It is a great thing to be consistent and true to the real Advent message (J.V. Himes to E.G. White, Mar.13; cf. Himes' further letter of Sept. 12, 1894 cited in Knight, 1995: 143).

Sectarian Isolation verses Social Concern

Adventism commenced its sectarian journey in considerable tension with its environment, with a number of significant differences distinguishing the movement from mainstream American Protestant denominations. The two most obvious were Sabbath observance and the expectation of the imminent, visible Advent of Christ to earth (both explicit in the movement's name, Seventh-day Adventist). Accompanying these two fundamental differences were a cluster of lifestyle issues that further encouraged the Adventist separatist stance. These included, dietary restrictions (including prohibitions on alcohol, coffee and tea); behavioral concerns (no gambling, dancing, card playing, reading of fictitious materials, theatre attendance, or smoking); a commitment to dress reform including abstinence from the use of makeup, jewelry adornment and a refusal to bear arms when conscripted (Lawson, 1998: 655).

From a theological perspective, Adventism identified itself as God's remnant people, the one truly unique vessel through which God would deliver His final proclamation of warning and rebuke to the world. Adventism's self-appraisal and separatist stance became transparent by its bold declarations that other contemporary religious groups were "apostate" and had succumbed to the "whore of Babylon." Its brazen challenges to clergy from other religious groups that were in collaboration with the state, all tended to create and foster bitter, mutually held antagonisms and were heightened and reinforced by the extent to which Adventism continued to physically separate from society (Lawson, 1998: 655).

The Millerite call for all true believers in the near Advent of Christ to separate and "come out of her my people" (i.e. out of the mainline Protestant churches) during the 1840s became the watchword. Millerite leaders began to identify and accuse the Protestant denominations of fulfilling the role of "Babylon" depicted in Revelation 14 and 18 for spurning the true Adventist message (Morgan, 2001: 12).

The year after the harrowing events of the Great Disappointment, on 22 October 1844 when their Lord did not return as predicted, a number of distressed and traumatized Millerite Advent believers (those who insisted that while the date remained correct, the nature of the expected event was incorrect) were still searching for answers and seeking a united course. They suffered, instead, further rejection at the hands of other former "mainline" Second Advent believers who repudiated their interpretation of 1844 by denying them an invitation to a specially convened Adventist conference (held in Albany, New York in 1845). Thus, within the space of a year, the spurned Millerite Adventists, who would eventually form the nucleus of future Seventh-day Adventism, "had been rejected not only by Protestantism at large but also by their fellow Adventists . . . They were the true Protestants rejected by the nominal churches, the true Adventists rejected by the nominal Adventists" (Morgan, 2001: 13).

Although the smallest of the splintered post Millerite Adventist groups, the rejected believers envisaged themselves as the true successors of all that was good in the previous Millerite movement. While these emerging Adventists knew where they stood in relation to Roman Catholicism, it now appeared equally obvious where they stood in relation to Protestantism. Isolated and despairing, the "true heirs" of the Millerite movement sought refuge and solace in the company of fellow travelers. Their lives centered on the faith, hope and fellowship of like believers, including a network of subcultures.

As time continued, their children increasingly attended church–sponsored schools; preferred employment was within church organizations and the majority of Adventists were frequently drawn by increasing educational opportunities and social and economic ties to reside in what became known colloquially as "New Jerusalems" or "Adventist Ghettos" (Lawson, 1998: 655). Adventists were essentially a community of outsiders, with their separatist stance strengthened by their theological interpretations, dietary and social prohibitions and prescribed behavior, which made members distinct and generally uncomfortable with those of other religious faiths or social persuasions.

Stepping into the present, it becomes apparent that the tension between Seventh-day Adventists and the surrounding societies has decreased significantly in many regions of the world. The development and accreditation of educational and medical institutions, in particular, coupled with commercially successful health food industries, has facilitated further participation in society and provided numerous opportunities for church members' upward mobility (Wilson, 1990: 51). During the last century, Adventist health care and medicine has become increasingly mainstream and orthodox, with denominational hospitals accorded recognition within their respective communities. The progression from a counter- establishment health reform movement to accepted mainstream medical institutions has proved decisive in providing overall upward mobility for the movement, whilst simultaneously diluting its sectarianism. If publishing endeavors instigated the need for SDA organization, the shift towards recognized medical practice exerted a profound impact on the nature of SDA organization, which has continued to gather momentum:

> This shift led, first, to a reorganized medical school, then to accreditation of colleges to feed the medical school, then to professional seminary education to keep the ministry apace with medicine . . . the blend of material and spiritual impulses which characterized mid-Victorianism played itself out in the movement, as Adventists came a long way, and rather quickly, from the sacrificial Millerites (Butler, 1993: 204).

The emergence of the regular five-day working week effectively removed the dilemma of Sabbath observance, while SDA dietary reforms and anti-smoking stance have netted increasing credibility in the eyes of governments and the general medical fraternity (Lawson, 1998). Contemporary Adventism has further diminished levels of antagonism with society by pursuing good relations with government departments through such humanitarian agencies as the Adventist Development and Relief Agency (ADRA). It is not uncommon today, particularly in urban regions, to observe a number of SDA congregations sharing their facilities with non-Adventist groups, providing further evidence that modern Adventism, in general, seeks to enhance rather than obstruct closer relationships with other religious traditions and society.

Early Adventists viewed the establishment and operation of institutions as an unnecessary distraction from preparation for the imminent Advent of Christ. White observed, however, that the Advent delay might be prolonged, suggesting that institution building was a necessary work to prepare for the Lord's coming:

> A great work must be done all through the world, and let no one conclude that, because the end is near, there is no need of special effort to build up the various institutions as the cause shall demand. . . . When the Lord shall bid us make no further effort to build meetinghouses and establish schools, sanitariums, and publishing houses, it will be time for us to fold our hands and let the Lord close up the work; but now is our opportunity to show zeal for God throughout the world; wherever there are souls to be saved, we are to lend our help, that many sons and daughters may be brought to God (6T: 440).

This developing ideological shift from imminent to delayed Advent brought in its wake the seeds of tension between sectarian isolation and social concern; between preaching and teaching imminence and "occupying till the Lord returns." Within twenty years of formal organisation, Adventists were simultaneously "creating a considerably isolated subculture and attempting to penetrate the larger society through evangelism" (VandeVere, 1986: 67). The training of Adventist physicians, colporteurs (literature evangelists), ministers and teachers in Adventist institutions for future work in the world resulted in ambiguity. The attempt to train and socialize Adventist young people in separate institutional settings for future evangelistic work directed largely at the operation of those same (health, educational, publishing, media) institutions, led to a discernible tension between sectarian isolation and increased concern with secular society (Vance, 1999: 69).

While the Seventh-day Sabbath and a number of other religious prescriptions have made social interaction with outsiders difficult, the development of SDA institutions has created communities in which Adventists feel comfortable in associating with fellow travelers. This "colonization" also serves to maintain a view of the world that is at odds with radical secularism (Bull, 1988: 155; Guy, 1972: 27). Vance's (1999: 69) conclusion concerning the Adventist dilemma is illuminating:

> In its attempt to build unique institutions conducive to sectarian separation and then to use those institutions to evangelise the world, [Adventism] became poised between two disparate ends . . . the means (institution building) adopted in the attempt to reach Adventism's desired end (successful evangelism) seemingly denied the movement's explicit raison d'etre (the parousia).

Theobald was equally accurate in assessing the tension within Adventism when declaring:

> For a movement which still formally commits itself to a belief in the imminent end of things . . . extensive this worldly involvement, particularly in institutions and activities which are directed to the preservation and improvement of mortal existence, would seem to pose something of a paradox (1985: 110).

Thus, Adventists, called to be in the world but not of, or tainted by the world, in their attempt to achieve their goal of spreading the gospel message throughout the earth, have often withdrawn from secular society into Adventist communities. In the process, they have developed numerous institutions and organizations to meet both temporal and religious needs. While on a theological level Adventists preach and teach about Christ's soon coming, a large number continue to invest in temporal education, participate in "worldly" occupations and the aggregation of wealth. The tensions resulting from these various conflicts have led to a number of specific identity crises in Adventism (Vance, 1999: 71).

In attempting to hold all this together across its comparatively brief history, the SDA church has witnessed the development of an extensive bureaucratic structure while continuing to perceive strong elements of charismatic authority in the person of Ellen White. Whereas early Adventism was marked by apocalyptic urgency declaring that the coming of

Christ and the "end of the world" were imminent, today the institutional stakes are embedded deeply in society, suggesting that "occupancy" has overtaken "imminence" as an Adventist priority. The continued lapse of time has witnessed the maturing fruits of secularization, medicalization and institutionalization, with expressions of an imminent *parousia* becoming increasingly muted.

Thus said, it is clear that a major dilemma facing Seventh-day Adventism today is whether temporal goals will displace future Advent goals. Adventists continue to insist that temporal work will "hasten the Advent" and so they continue to utilize institutions in the hope of sharing the news about Christ's coming. Adventist institutionalism has simultaneously created space and justification for Adventist separation from secular society while at the same time it has lessened Adventist distinctiveness from the world (Vance, 1991: 70). These continuing tensions have brought into question and challenged the *identity* of the SDA movement.

Prior to examining the contribution of and disparities between Ellen White and Dr. Kellogg's understanding of the medical missionary vocation in Adventism, a contextualization of health reform activity in the 19th century is required.

2

Contextualizing Health Reform
in Nineteenth-Century America

THE NOVEMBER 2005 EDITION of the *National Geographic* featured an article titled, 'The Secrets of Long Life,' funded in part by the U.S. National Institute on Aging. Scientists focused on three regions of the world where people live significantly longer, produce a higher rate of centenarians, suffer a fraction of the diseases that commonly threaten people elsewhere and enjoy more healthy years of life overall. The three regions included the islands of Okinawa, Japan where longevity is among the highest on earth; the mountain villages of Sardinia, Italy where males reach age 100 regularly, and finally in Loma Linda, CA, researchers studied a group of Seventh-day Adventists who rank among America's longevity all-stars (Buettner, 2005).

Interestingly, Seventh-day Adventism portrays two differing images to the world. The first image could be labelled 'apocalyptic urgency' stretching back from the post Millerite years to the present. This image involves a religious movement whose fundamental premise is to preach, teach and evangelise the world concerning the imminent, premillennial return of Christ to earth; a message of both warning and judgment that insists probation for all humankind will soon terminate. The majority of Adventists continue to insist that their earthly duration and occupation is for the sole purpose of spreading the gospel and once complete, the Lord will return. Not unlike the Millerites, Adventists are often depicted and portrayed as adherents of a religious organization expressed in lurid, apocalyptic symbols (Bull & Lockhart, 2007: 8). Thus, for many Adventists, this present world is a mere 'stepping stone' to the eventual heavenly realm.

Bull & Lockhart also insist that an alternative image of the SDA church exists, and this representation is almost completely at odds with the apocalyptic imagery, and subtle hints of this alternative image are clearly evident in the responses provided to public perception surveys, noted in the previous chapter, which indicated that a minimal number of people are actually aware that Adventists are unusually concerned with the end of this world (2007: 11).

What emerged clearly in the 2003 poll, however, was the public's strong association of Adventists with health. Of those who were aware of Adventism, 19% were acquainted with the health-orientated Adventist television program *Lifestyle Magazine*, hosted by the Adventist actor Clifton Davis. More than 6% knew of an Adventist medical center in their community, and 4% stated that they or a relative had been cared for in an Adventist hospital. "Such activities," the authors note, "are very different from the other-worldly obsessions often thought to characterize the church." Indeed, Adventist lifestyle and practices are seen as being concerned not with the end of life on the planet but with its improvement, that is, a 'this-worldly' emphasis (Bull & Lockhart, 2007: 11).

It was also noted previously that nineteenth century America experienced a multitude of converging changes built upon rapid progress. Unprecedented geographical expansion, accompanied by a powerful and fervent nationalistic spirit was evident (Damsteegt, 1977: 4), simultaneously overlapping with a groundswell in religious plurality and diversity with successful and established denominations experiencing the tensions and pressures associated with new religious boundaries, particularly as new sects proliferated. The population at the turn of the century was only 5 million, however, by the 1850s that figure had risen to 25 million (Mayfield, 1982: 6).

Gaustad (1974: xv) declares that a new climate of enthusiasm was celebrated by revivalists and millennialists, utopians and communitarians, spiritualists and prophesiers, polygamists and celibates, perfectionists and transcendentalists—they were all present and very active. Ferret, in a similar vein, argues that the increasing optimism of revival fueled by significant changes taking place in American society after 1814 provided fertile soil for a multitude of reform movements across the nation. Furthermore, the burgeoning territorial expansion coincided with improved living standards and the transition from an elitist to a somewhat democratic political landscape were all taking place with such rapidity that many Americans felt that life was spiraling out of control (2008: 37). In response, multitudes engaged in movements to institute temperance ideals, establish humane treatment of debtors and the insane, improve health and take education to the masses and most importantly, to end slavery (Dick, 1986: 6). The predominant values of individualism and liberty influenced all spheres of existence and challenged to the core traditional religious authority and moral life (Hatch, 1989). Both sectarianism and denominationalism proliferated (Jackson, 2015: 138).

Religion, Politics and Reform Mania

The reform mania or 'ultraism' endemic across the American landscape was based on the post-millennium assumption that only the total moral regeneration of humankind could, in fact, inaugurate the millennium. Thus, according to Theobald, all social and individual imperfections were obstacles to its realization, and as such, must be eradicated (1979: 24). This was the major ethos that spawned postmillennialism.

The majority of Americans living during the antebellum period agreed with the optimistic postmillennial interpretation of the prophecies of Revelation, and following in the established tradition of Jonathan Edwards and company, that Christ's Second Advent would occur only after peace and prosperity had been achieved on earth through the agency of human beings (Wilson, 2014: 5). Indeed, the majority of American Christians not only believed, but fully expected that they could cooperate alongside other citizens of the United States to cultivate a form of social and political existence which would not only realize the Enlightenment ideals, but consummate humanity's elusive dreams for love, justice, compassionate relationships, purity of intention, among all economic and economic classes (Smith, 1974: 19). Thus, many Americans firmly believed that their homeland could soon become the ideal society in which the major forms of social evil would be eliminated (Reid, 1982: 53). This millennial impulse became the focus of intense anticipation and rabid speculation through revivalist preaching and reform programs (Damsteegt, 1977: 7).

Andrew Johnson, one of General Andrew Jackson's most committed supporters, who was inaugurated President in 1829, ardently believed that humanity was capable of elevating itself to the realm of divinity. "Let us go on elevating our people and perfecting our institutions," Johnson declared, "until democracy shall reach such a point of perfection that we can acclaim with truth that voice of the people is the voice of God" (Hudson, 1974: 2). This new perspective and process became known as the 'era of the common man' and Jackson's election to Presidency sparked the imagination of the ordinary American, leading to innovation, and experimentation fueled by optimism (Jackson, 2015: 137). Johnson's views concerning the grandeur of this new religious and political marriage were no more evident than in the following quote:

> The democratic party proper of the whole world, and especially of the United States, has undertaken the *political redemption of man*, and sooner or later the great work will be accomplished. In the political world it corresponds to that of Christianity in the moral. They are going along, not in divergents nor in parallels, but in converging lines—the one purifying and elevating man religiously, the other politically . . . at what period of time they will have finished the work of progress and elevation is not now to determine, but when finished these two lines will have approximated each other-man being perfected both in a religious and a political point of view (Hudson, 1974: 1, 2).

The thought of a new national utopia of reforms appealed to and excited many through a democratizing process (Reynolds, 2008: 87). Finally, the proclamation could ring out through the nation that the millennial dawn was on the horizon and in classic biblical language from the book of Revelation; the lion and lamb would lie down together. Thus, the joyful tidings will be proclaimed on earth that humanity's political and religious redemption is complete and that peace on earth and good will towards men will be universally inaugurated (Hudson, 1974: 2, 3). This enveloping creed was a "curious blend of faith in the efficacy of democratic institutions and evangelical religion to perfect the individual and thus perfect society" (Hudson, 1974: 2, 3). These ideals would become significant in the development of health reform movements for moral action and holiness undergirded by post-millennial hopes led to a renewed emphasis on transforming society through organized voluntary agencies. Nathan Hatch (1989) argues that the role of Christian revivals and their membership in voluntary societies contributed significantly to ensuing American democracy. Many Christians believed that they could play a pivotal role in the eradication of societal ills including prostitution, alcoholism, poverty and slavery. The impact of the religious impulse on society was very tangible (Jackson, 2015; 139).

For the Millerite believers, however, it was of no consequence, for they sincerely believed the complete opposite—that is, mankind was not on a progressively upward journey, rather, humanity was on a spiraling, downward course, and only the literal, visible premillennial return of Christ to earth would bring an end to all evil and worldly matters and usher in the kingdom of God. While the post-millennial impulse was heightened by the success of the Revolutionary War and the founding of the American Republic, premillennial interpretations were once again voiced in response to the repulsion of the French Revolution in Europe that echoed across the Atlantic.

The American homeland was also experiencing changing attitudes with the combination of religious fervor and excitement generated by the Second Great Awakening coinciding with the social dislocation as a result of the War in 1812. Both scenarios provided fruitful soil in which renewed growth of premillennialist ideas could flourish and which became the theological foundation on which the future Seventh-day Adventist theological edifice would be constructed (Wilson, 2014: 5).

Ferret (2008: 45) declares that for the majority of Americans at this time, the core of acceptable belief posited the divine who functioned within and through people and their institutions, not through a cataclysmic, literal Advent of Christ into their world. Indeed, it was this concept of 'radical supernaturalism' of God literally intervening in the affairs of humanity on earth that was the defining differentiation distinguishing Millerism from American Protestantism (Doan, 1987: 54, 82, 198).

Medical Folklore and the Age of Quackery

Paul Starr provides an overview of early to mid-nineteenth century medical practice suggesting that health matters was shared by three groups: domesticated women, regular physicians, and those engaged in popular medicine (1982: Location 1060). The prevailing social conditions in America meant that the bulk of medical care was provided for by women in the home. It was expected that women would acquire a basic knowledge of how to treat common disorders and apply traditional remedies (Starr, 1982: Location, 949). Their knowledge and skills were largely dependent on prior experience, experimentation and oral tradition. Furthermore, the ongoing transformation of politics and religion that gave voice to the common and often uneducated people was accompanied by simple home health care guides authored by physicians who were skeptical and critical of those who sought to control medical knowledge. A popular example was *Domestic Medicine*, written by William Buchanan that stressed the importance of moderation in diet, fresh air, cleanliness, avoidance of liquor and strong spices etc. (Jackson, 2014: 140).

Mainstream or Allopathic medicine began to emerge as a professional group in the mid-nineteenth century. Initial education was gained through an apprenticeship model, and by 1850, forty-two medical schools were operating. It cannot be assumed, however, that medical practice improved substantially. Most medical courses consisted of three or four months duration with laboratory and practical experiences quite rare (Agnew, 2010: 20). Common treatments included bloodletting, the application of leeches, purging, vomiting along with drugs such as nux vomica (strychnine), calomel (a mercury-based laxative) and opium products. Blake suggests that many physicians at the time recognized despairingly that their current treatments were largely unsuccessful but were simultaneously hindered from progressing by a lack of viable treatment options, resulting in a third group who provided medical care by embracing the ideas of popular medicine, particularly if they were associated with natural laws (1974: 35).

Popular medicine advocates were afforded credence due to the enthusiasm of the populace for simple remedies that worked and were freely available, and by the failure of allopathic medicine (Jackson, 2015: 141). Medicine practitioners tended to rely on natural remedies that emphasized natural laws (vegetarian diet, exercise, fresh air, opposition to alcohol, tobacco, tea etc.). Their popularity grew immensely and they soon rivalled trained physicians in society (Starr, 1982, locations 1269, 1347).

Homeopathy and hydrotherapy found their niche in this environment, particularly as the public were loathe to continue with failed treatments and their debilitating side effects (Blake, 1974: 34). Jackson argues that popular medicine consisted of an eclectic combination of various approaches to health, and it was common for practitioners to blend a number of these elements in their treatment regime (2015: 142).

In tracing the development of Adventism's alternative image (health orientation) as previously noted by Bull & Lockhart, Ronald Numbers, a specialist in American health reform, sets the scene vividly when describing the period's general health habits:

For all its apparent vitality, America in the early nineteenth century was a sick and dirty nation. Public sanitation was grossly inadequate and personal hygiene, virtually nonexistent. The great majority of Americans seldom, if ever, bathed. Their eating habits, including the consumption of gargantuan amounts of meat, were enough to keep most stomachs continually upset. Fruits and green leafy vegetables seldom appeared on the table, and the food that did appear was often saturated with butter or lard. A 'common' breakfast consisted of 'Hot bread, made with lard and strong alkalies, and soaked with butter; hot griddle cakes, covered with butter and syrup; meats fried in fat or baked in it; potatoes dripping with grease; ham and eggs fried in grease into a leathery indigestibility—all washed down with many cups of strong Brazil coffee (2008: 95).

In the spirit of true Jacksonianism, the common man became the expert. The American Medical Association organized in 1847 was powerless to regulate medical education or practice. Freedom prevailed to the point that anyone with an assortment of drugs or a casual interest in health and healing could practice medicine (Schaefer, 2005: 74). Relatively few Americans lived long enough during this period to suffer from the many degenerative organic diseases that threaten their descendants today. Tuberculosis was the chief killer at that time, not twenty-first-century heart disease.

Individuals were also quite likely to discover that their longevity was endangered by a plethora of other illnesses including cholera, pneumonia, yellow fever, malaria and typhoid. Less likely to prove fatal but nonetheless both common and debilitating were dyspepsia, catarrh, rheumatism and asthma. Such was the prevalence of impaired digestion that one writer called dyspepsia "the great endemic of the northern states" (Martin, 1942: 45–46, 74–76).

Homemade concocted remedies were commonplace and folk would rather dose themselves with their favorite Indian cure or herbal tea, than consult a physician. The more bizarre its components, and the more bitter tasting the home remedy, declares Schwarz, the more highly it was esteemed (2006: 21). A. W. Spaulding in the first volume of the *Origin and History of Seventh-day Adventists* might well have provided the best summation of those pre-health reform conditions when declaring:

> The days of our fathers were days of many afflictions. They were smitten with sore diseases, described as lung fever, typhoid. Cholera, catarrh. . . . For relief their physicians gave them strychnine,

mercury, opium, alcohol, and tobacco. They forbade them water internally or externally, and bled them. . . . Baths were accounted hazardous, the weekly wash-off in the wooden tub by the kitchen stove [was] . . . reckoned a part of unnecessary sorrows. . . . The diet was heavy laden with meats filled with hot spices. On the frontier it was washed down with cider or whiskey and in the East with tea and coffee. No one—almost no one—saw any relationship between this diet and the ills of the flesh they endured. . . . All these were visitations of an inscrutable Providence, intended to torment the wicked and to perfect the saints for an early entrance into Paradise (335, 336).

Folk had significant reason, however, to be suspicious of early nineteenth-century medical practitioners. An apprenticeship under the supervision of another physician was often the only requirement for gaining approval to practice medicine. Minimal, if any clinical training was required and attendance at a formal course of lectures was encouraged but not mandatory, while medical schools, library facilities and laboratories were in their infancy. In spite of doctors in Europe during the 1930s, providing significant evidence displaying the futility of such procedures, the standardized procedure for the treatment of disease in America consisted almost entirely on purging, bleeding, and polypharmacy (Reid, 1982: 21) Drugs were as equally plentiful as were their varied dosages prescribed. Trial and error became the norm of the day. Thus, if one drug did not appear to work, another was tried, and so on until the patient expired, recovered, or decided to endure their malady. Calomel became such a favorite purgative that folk spoke of pioneer farmers as living on calomel and bread (Schwarz, 2006: 22).

Quackery also flourished at this time, so much so, Orestes A. Brownson in a university address at the time, made the poignant observation regarding 'quackeries' pervasiveness:

The age in which we live is the age of quackery. We are overrun with quackery, with quackery, with quackery of every description. I refer not merely to quack medicines, which, though bad enough in all conscience, are by no means the worst or most deleterious species of quackery with which we are infested. We have quack economics, quack politics, quack law, quack learning, and quack divinity; quackery everywhere, and sometimes one, in a fit of despair or spleen, fancies nowhere anything but quackery (Reid, 1982: 35).

A brief perusal of recommended treatments for prevailing ailments at the time reveal a plethora of medical folklore options, some of which are as follows:

- Tobacco was recommended for any lung problem, the vapor to be produced by smoking a cigar. To achieve the greatest benefit the patient should frequently draw in the breath freely, so that the internal surface of the air vessels may be exposed to the action of the vapor).

- To treat an earache: blow the smoke of tobacco strongly into the affected ear.

- To cure baldness: rub the head morning and evening, first with onions until the head is red and then with honey.

- To treat worms: patient must swallow a teaspoon of molasses mixed with a teaspoon of tin rust.

- To stop a nosebleed: patient must chew a newspaper, or hold a dime on the roof of the mouth with the tongue for a few minutes, or wrap the little finger with thread (Schaefer, 2005: 77).

The cause of actual diseases were essentially conjecture with the majority of the Christianized world deeming suffering and illness a result of divine infliction alleviated, if possible, through prayer and faith (Douglass, 1998: 279). Human longevity was reduced on average to 39.4 years as both ignorance and confusion took center stage concerning medical matters with supposed orthodox medicine and quackery operating together simultaneously, with both mixing a portion of truth with large doses of unadulterated nonsense (Coon, 1993: 12). The medical treatment slogan was characterized by the four Ps—purge, puke, plaster, and poison (Coon, 1993: 11). The enveloping new focus on the individual and simultaneous departure from traditional theories was increasingly apparent in the burgeoning concerns for personal health (Bull & Lockhart, 2007: 162–164). This resulted in a fundamental distrust of traditional medicine with its so called 'heroic' treatments and pitiful results and, eventuating in turning the minds of many from all classes of society to examine what might be achieved with a good dose of 'common sense!' (Schoepflin: 1987: 143–158).

The theme of health reform was, therefore, a broadly discussed topic in the world in which the Millerites inhabited. Since the 1820s, many Americans had been endorsing and promoting an assortment of social reforms, most prominently the abolition of slavery, but also included were new methods of treating the handicapped, insane, poor, criminals, and the advocacy of women's rights, popular education, world peace, and health and temperance reforms (Schwarz, 2006: 21). It has been suggested that the Millerite millennialist expectation was the spiritual counterpart of the physical reforms of the era, which, as noted in the previous quote, included health reform (Whorton, 1982: 59). This health impetus was assisted by the increasing distrust of the professionals, elite and intellectuals in society and the health reformers, who advocated prevention rather than cure (Willis, 2003: 21), and found both receptive and fertile minds as the enveloping mood described as the "rise of the common man" gained momentum (Craig, 1991: 35).

A number of alternative treatment regimens arose at the time, collectively known as 'sectarian medicine', which emphasized the 'healing power of nature.' Sectarian medicine was far more concerned with prevention than with cure and its focus and methods were largely built on balancing the six Galenic 'non-naturals', including: air, diet, sleeping and waking, exercise and rest, evacuations, and peace of mind. Sectarian health reformers believed that whilst moral sins lead to spiritual diseases, it was 'physiological sins' that were responsible for bodily diseases. The implications were obvious: if spiritual diseases could be avoided by following the moral code (Ten Commandments), so too could physiological sins be avoided by observing the 'laws of life' (Wilson, 2014: 14). Some reformers rose to great prominence, and exerted a wider influence than others, particularly influencing the development of Kellogg's health reform agenda and resonating with future Adventist health reforms.

The initial sporadic attempts to re-educate the American populace concerning health reform commenced in the 1830s, led by the controversial and egotistical Sylvester Graham, who was both an evangelist and health reform advocate (Numbers, 2008: 97). Throughout the 1830s, Graham, inventor of what became known as the famous 'Graham Cracker', lectured on the benefits of temperance and vegetarianism, with the most distinctive of his ideas concerned with dietary practices.

The best way to maintain health, argued Graham, was to avoid all unnatural and stimulating foods and to survive entirely on the produce from the vegetable kingdom and pure water, which he argued, was the only fluid that man can ever consume in perfect harmony with the essential properties and laws of his nature (Numbers, 2008: 99). There was, however, an underlying emphasis, and one that Grahamism shared with a number of health reformers—a moral and religious foundation undergirded true health reform. Medicine had consistently been enveloped with a religious aura, no more so than the early nineteenth-century health reform movement, which were propelled forward, in part, by the energies overflowing from the period's fervent evangelical pietism, and further inspired by the Christian perfectionism of Charles Finney (Wilson, 2014: 16).

Dr. Joel Shew's *Water Cure Journal*, published in 1845 was deemed helpful by many, particularly after the facile pen of Russell T. Trall began to promote and endorse the wonders of hydrotherapy (Schwarz, 1979: 104, 105). Changing attitudes were evident by the time Horace Mann in the early 1840s wrote that suffering was not a part of merciful providence but is a direct result of human ignorance and error. Furthermore, if people would simply observe God's original physical laws, they would no more suffer pain than they would suffer moral pain or remorse, if in all things they would continue to obey God's moral laws (Reid, 1982, 21).

Dr. L. B. Coles of Boston published his *Philosophy of Health* in 1848 in which he presented simple rules for healthful living that could be understood by the general populace. While including all the major health reform concepts by the earlier reformers, Coles placed special emphasis on humanities moral duty to observe and obey the laws governing healthful living, and furthermore, failure to keep the laws of health was regarded as being as sinful as breaking the Ten Commandments (Schwarz, 2006: 26). In other words, both spiritual and physiological sins affect one's salvation. Thus Coles could declare, "it is as truly a duty to read and be informed on the subject [of health], as it is to study the precepts of the Bible." The study of the Bible should come first, and the study of the laws of life next because the natural laws are directly connected with the path that leads to heaven (Damsteegt, 1978: 14, 16).

Wilson argues that when the American Physiological Association (APA) was founded in 1837, more than one's personal salvation was at stake as far as health reform was concerned (2014: 16, 17). The APA emphasized the importance of yielding a firm obedience to the natural laws, as part of the grand system of God, asserting that the impending millennium, so confidently predicted, can never be expected to arrive until those laws which God has implanted in the physical nature of man are considered equal with his moral laws, and universally obeyed (Blake, 1974: 43).

William Alcott, a contemporary of Graham also called for a reformed diet and reliance on exercise, bathing, rest, and the abandonment of tea, alcohol, and coffee to improve health (Schwarz, 1979, 104). Alcott purposed to consume only water and milk, repudiated meat, fish and all stimulants, and his diet consisted mainly of vegetables (Willis, 2003: 21). Alcott became the first president of APA and authored over 100 journals and books on health reform. He was also a self-styled medical missionary, medical prophet and chief rival of Sylvester Graham, who deemed it his duty to educate the American public concerning the laws of hygiene as "a means of lifting us toward the Eden whence we came." By observing the physiological laws, humans could once again experience perfect health, the total elimination of disease, and a lifespan consistent with the antediluvians, ultimately elevating the human race over time to a place of perfection. All of which resonates with the postmillennialism position predicted by the APA (Wilson, 2014: 17). Perhaps Alcott voiced the religious and millennial aspects of sectarian health best with his designated millennial brand of health reform labelled 'Christian Physiology,' a philosophy which situates physiology as the cornerstone and foundation of the earthly kingdom (Wilson, 2014: 17).

By the mid-1840s, whilst considerable headway had been achieved concerning a comprehensive system for maintaining good health, the same cannot be said for the restoration of health once it was forfeited. A number of reform enterprises arose in response to what was deemed the antiquated practices of bleeding, purging and blistering associated with so-called conventional medical practice. These safer-sectarian systems included among others, Thomsonianism, and homeopathy, or hydrotherapy. Samuel Thomson, a New Hampshire farmer and founder of the Thomsonian medical sect, prescribed 'natural' botanic remedies instead of the regularly prescribed drug concoctions by regular physicians. Thomson's became convinced that all disease resulted from a cold environment, and that the only cure was to restore normal body temperature, which was achieved primarily by the application of steaming, peppering and puking patients with large doses of lobelia, an emetic used by the Native Americans. Thomson patented his practice in 1813, but by the 1840s, internal issues fragmented the movement and as botanic strength began to decline, yet another new sect, homeopathy, rose to national prominence.

Instead of the regular bleedings, purging and drug therapy of conventional medical practices, homeopathy, instead, offered pleasant-tasting pills that apparently produced no discomforting or lingering side effects, and the same medication was suitable for babies and small children

(Numbers, 2008: 112, 113). It was perhaps the later reason, more than any other, which won widespread support throughout the nation. Numbers argues that while Thomsonianism and homeopathy attracted some health reformers, ultimately the majority of health reformers distrusted all medicines, whether in large or small doses, botanical or mineral. Instead, the majority of them opted for the one system of therapeutics that offered healing without drugs: hydrotherapy (2008: 113).

Dr. James Caleb Jackson, born in 1811, was arguably the most successful entrepreneur of the many 'water-cure' or hydropathic institutions that sprang up during the 1850s, and along with his adopted daughter, the Jacksons' also played a significant role in the dress reform movement. The entrepreneurial Dr. Jackson developed Granula, which became the first successful cold breakfast cereal produced in the early 1860s (Schwarz, 2006: 27). Jackson's early childhood was plagued by ill health and lack of education, the latter as a result of having to care for the family farm following his father's untimely death. Jackson often dreamed of another life away from the farm that would include public speaking and at 23 his aspirations were realized when he received invitations from nearby communities to speak on slavery and temperance matters. Once again, however, his frail constitution suffered under the load of increasing demands experienced on the speaking circuit and he opted to relinquish that role for a more sedate vocation editing antislavery papers and serving as secretary to abolitionist societies and organizations. When Jackson's health deteriorated to the point of death in 1847, a colleague encouraged him to attend Dr. Silas Gleason's water cure facility in Cuba, New York. Jackson not only survived the ordeal despite the harsh water treatment endured, but his improvement in health was accompanied by a heightened interest in hydrotherapy, eventually resulting in the establishment of 'Our Home on the Hillside' in Dansville, New York (Numbers, 2008: 121, 126).

Essentially, hydrotherapy, which originated in Austria under the auspices of Vincent Priessnitz, endeavored to cure people through the copious application of fresh water, taken either internally or externally through baths, showers, or wet-blanket wraps (Wilson, 2014: 17). In an atmosphere similar to the European health spa, Jackson provided hydropathic treatments coupled with a special diet for up to 1,000 patients a year. Russell Trall, who along with Joel Shew, opened the first hydropathic facility in the United States, wrote in his *Water-Cure Journal*, "Health reform . . . is the veritable corner stone upon which the Christian, the social, the political, as well as the medical reformer must predicate all rational faith in the millennial state of the human family on this earth" (Wilson, 2014: 18). Indeed, Dr. Jackson's summation of the water-cure therapy was magnanimous to say the least when insisting that the water-cure revolution is a *great* revolution for it "touches more interests than any revolution since the days of Jesus Christ" (Numbers, 2008: 95).

While the majority of health reformers attempted to keep their egos intact, and as such could not find consensus on every aspect of each other theories, preferring to believe that their particular theory was both original and correct, they did stress the following core teachings: diet reform, regular exercise, avoidance of stimulating drinks, eradication of tobacco use, electrotherapy, increased use of water, good ventilation and sanitation, and the use of herbal or natural remedies (Willis, 2003: 21). Of more significance, sectarian health reform sought to reconnect physical health with spiritual health, that is, physiological disease with moral or spiritual decay. It was a millennialist reform movement titled, 'Christian Physiology' where the books of revelation and of nature, emanate from the hand of the same author, and as such, must be considered mutually reinforcing (Wilson, 2014: 16).

Early Evidence of Adventist Health Reform

Although some Sabbatarian Adventists remained sympathetic to health reform following the Great Disappointment of 1844, the more pressing question of the pre-millennialist, Second Advent of Christ continued to remain uppermost in their minds for several years. Schwarz provides a succinct rationale declaring that early Sabbatarian Adventists were not interested in the virtues of vegetarianism, cold and hot water packs, sunshine, and exercise. Rather, they were consumed with proclaiming the imminence of the advent, studying the prophecies of Daniel and the Revelation, and groping their way toward a formal organization (1979: 105).

While many Seventh-day Adventists assume that Ellen White inaugurated a health reform stance within the movement, it was another pioneer, Joseph Bates who discovered the value of altered habits in promoting health well before he joined the Millerite ranks (Knight, 2004: 200). It was during his career as a ship captain that Bates began to ponder the question of health reform more seriously and began abandoning practices he deemed harmful to both health and the moral character (Douglass, 1998: 280). In 1821, he discarded strong liquor, the following year wine was eradicated from his dining table and shortly thereafter tobacco was eliminated from his lifestyle habits, all of which took place prior to his conversion to Christ and admission to the Fairhaven, Massachusetts, Christian church. Bates' passion for health reform witnessed his involvement in organizing a local temperance society, and a decade before joining the Millerite movement, Bates eliminated both tea and coffee from his diet. As 1844, the year of Christ's expected return to earth came into sharp focus, Bates modified his diet even more drastically. Eliminated from the pantry, table and personal consumption on this occasion were the use of meat, cheese, butter, pies, grease, and rich cakes. Such was his passion for reform; by 1845, Bates diet consisted almost entirely of bread and water alone. A slight compromise, re-modification or balance in dietary practice occurred a little later with the inclusion of fruits, vegetables, cereals and nuts. Evidently, the former sea captain's health improved considerably in contrast to many other Adventist leaders and members who were frequently plagued with poor health. While Joseph Bates was a staunch Millerite believer and later, a devoted and energetic pioneer of the Sabbatarian Adventist movement, which included his convincing James and Ellen White of the integrity of the Sabbath of the fourth commandment, he was not a "health-reforming evangelist" nor did he seek to persuade others of the same (Douglass, 1998: 280). Interestingly, Bates made no point of advancing his dietary practices until after Ellen White received her health visions, nonetheless, his quiet witness and demeanor must have impressed his associates (Schwarz, 1979, 105, 106).

The Sabbatarian Adventists, based on Ellen White's instruction, began to reluctantly contemplate an earthly sojourn that was now required to balance Advent immediacy with earthly occupation, a tension foreign to their Millerite forebears. An essential part of the future SDA earthly sojourn would encompass a developing awareness of health reform principles. It was White, therefore, who was primarily responsible for establishing a direct link between Seventh-day Adventism and health (Jackson, 2015: 147).

As early as 1848, White was also shown the harmful effects of tobacco, coffee and tea, which complimented Bate's prior position. A number of the Sabbatarian believers, however, were not easily convinced of this new health impetus and challenged the young pioneer. In a letter penned in 1851, White wrote, "I have seen in vision that tobacco was a filthy weed, and it must be laid aside or given up" (1 Bio: 224). Other health issues including dietary practice (particularly the consumption of pork), lifestyle changes, cleanliness, health maintenance, etc., continued to be zealously debated among the Adventist believers for some years. Prior to the early battle against tea, coffee and tobacco being won, White began to broaden her appeal for Adventists to make appropriates changes to improve their health (Schwarz, 1979: 106), for Sabbath keepers were to display a higher standard of cleanliness than was currently evident (EW, 1854: Manuscript 1).

It was not, however, until White's epochal health vision on June 6, 1863, a mere two weeks following formal church organization that the subject of health reform became an integral part of the early Seventh-day Adventist agenda. James White, in a reflective moment, in 1870, contextualized his wife's health message:

> The Lord also knew how to introduce to His waiting people the great subject of health reform, step by step, so they could bear it, and make a good use of it, without souring the public mind. It was twenty-two years ago [1848] . . . that our minds were called to the injurious effects of tobacco, tea, and coffee, through the testimony of Mrs. White. God has wonderfully blessed the effort to put these things away from us, so that we as a denomination can rejoice in victory, with very few exceptions, over these pernicious indulgences of appetite. . . . When we had gained a good victory over these things, and when the Lord saw that we were able to bear it, light was given relative to food and dress (RH: May 27, 1902).

Wilson's insightful analysis recognizes that while White had on previous occasions spoken on several aspects of health reform, the Otsego revelation made it abundantly obvious that health reform should now become an integral part of the church and take its place among the other teachings of Adventism such as the sanctuary doctrine of atonement and the observance of Saturday worship (2014: 26). Following the Otsego vison in 1863, health reform became a significant seam in the developing SDA theological garment, so much so, that the health message was considered a pivotal aspect of the proclamation of the gospel in the context of the imminent return of Christ, or as White would coin the phrase, as close as the "hand is with the body" (3T: 62).

Several of the new health reform concepts received in vision astonished White and she wrote that many things came directly across her own ideas (3SM: 281). If the prescriptions of White's Otsego vision in 1863 offered little that had not previously been advocated, what is remarkable about her contribution is the manner in which it casts the "entirety of salvation history in terms of health reform" (Wilson, 2014: 27). Her motivations were based on her understanding of the link between health and spiritual experience. Essentially, and pragmatically, since human minds and bodies form the medium through which God communicates with individuals, truth can be better determined by healthy bodies. Furthermore, as the body is the temple of God it should be maintained in the purest condition possible (MH: 130). Healthy minds and bodies enabled better choices, clearer thought and thus the ability to serve God more effectively (MS 6a). Accomplishing God's purposes both as a church and as individuals were clearly dependent upon good health (Jackson, 2015: 148).

Contemporary Christian physiologists, as has been previously noted, also cited the scriptures in abundance regarding the merging of the physical and the spiritual in preparation for the millennium, however, White provided a distinctly Adventist insight when she wrote in 1867:

> God's people are not prepared for the loud cry of the third angel. They have a work to do for themselves which they should not leave for God to do for them. . . . Lustful appetite makes slaves of men and women, and beclouds their intellects and stupefies their moral sensibilities to such a degree that the sacred, elevated truths of God's Word are not appreciated. . . . In order to be fitted for translation, the people of God must know themselves. . . . They should ever have the appetite in subjection to the moral and intellectual organs (CDF: 32, 33).

In a real sense, the connection between the Second Advent and the Adventist church was inaugurated on the day the movement was birthed—October 22, 1844. Adventist eschatology has changed over time, but not the end-time role of Adventist believers. The ultimate separation from worldly conspiracies involving a counterfeit day of worship has provided a barrier between Adventists and society. "Yet," argues Bull & Lockhart, "the timing of the Second Advent is understood to be in the control of the movement called upon to await it." That is, the gospel must be preached throughout the world while simultaneously the Adventist believers must be perfect in readiness for heaven, for the Second Advent of Christ will take place only when Adventists have fulfilled the gospel commission and realized God's perfect ideals (2007: 68). Health reform for White, therefore, was a central component in realizing God's perfect ideals for His people. Thus, a belief in the imminent, pre-millennialist Advent of Christ in connection with a health reform emphasis was the major theological differential between her and other contemporary health reformers.

The vision Ellen White experienced in Rochester, New York on December 25, 1865 complimented the 1863 Otsego vision. White writes, "I was shown that there is a much greater work before us than we as yet have any idea of, if we would insure health by placing ourselves in the right relation to life . . . Our faith requires us to elevate the standard and take advance steps (1 T: 486–488). Those steps required an successful campaign of education in the principles of health reform to be established, and furthermore, a way had to be found for those who required medical attention to go to facilities where they could "not only receive rational treatment, but also be free from the temptation to violate their conscience" (Robinson, 1965: 141). Such was the immediate need for Adventists to develop their own institution that just three years later the Western Health Reform Institute in Michigan was opened by the SDA church in an effort to apply the principles of health reform in an institutional setting. Interestingly, White reluctantly complied with this new development as her concerns over the introduction of worldly themes and amusements as witnessed at the water cure institution under the leadership of Dr. Jackson in Dansville, New York were still uppermost in her mind. She also knew that several other hygienic institutions had enjoyed initial success only to experience ultimate failure (Schwarz, 1979: 113).

This sectarian impulse to remain separated, as far as humanly possible, from other non-Adventist institutions and organizations has been a veritable 'thorn in the flesh' of Adventism since its inception, particularly in relation to health and educational institutions. This tension was exacerbated between J. H. Kellogg, church ministers, administrators and White during the late 1800s and early twentieth century. A point often remiss by those studying religious movements is the impact that institutionalization effects on those same movements, particularly those birthed from sectarian roots. Crow (1993: 1) articulated the dilemma well:

> Institutionalization is necessary of religious movements but also detrimental to those movements . . . therefore . . . an analysis of the effects of institutionalization should observe not only what it does for the church but also what it does to the church.

In 1876 a young Adventist doctor, John Harvey Kellogg, was appointed medical director of the Western Health Reform Institute which within a few months he renamed the Battle Creek Sanitarium. The rationale for the name change was provided by Kellogg stating that the word *sanitarium*, would signify a "place where people learn to stay well" (Schwarz, 1979: 116). Both James and Ellen White were pleased with the appointment of Kellogg to direct the new health venture, for in the young Dr J. H. Kellogg they had found a resourceful and vigorous advocate to take the lead in transforming Adventist habits and spreading the health reform gospel to the world. Such was their confidence they felt they could now turn their attention to other lines of church endeavors that required attention (Schwarz, 1979: 116). From that time onward, the development of Adventism's interest in health was largely Kellogg's responsibility.

In 1897 Dr. Kellogg spoke to the assembled delegates at the General Conference session of Seventh-day Adventists concerning the invaluable contribution White's writings contributed to health reform, declaring:

> It is impossible for any man who has not made a special study of medicine to appreciate the wonderful character of instruction that has been received in these writings. It is wonderful brethren, when you look back over the writings that were given us thirty years ago, and then perhaps the next day pick up a scientific journal and find some new discovery that the microscope has made, or that has been brought to light in the chemical laboratory—I say, it is perfectly wonderful how correctly they agree in fact. . . . There is not a single principle in relation to the healthful development of our bodies and minds that is advocated in these writings from Sister White, which I am not prepared to demonstrate conclusively from scientific evidence (*General Conference Daily Bulletin*, March 8, 1897: 309; cited in Robinson, 1965: 84).

Two years later in March 1899 during another General Conference session convened in South Lancaster, Massachusetts the ministers of the Seventh-day Adventist church were strongly encouraged to support wholeheartedly the health principles, making them a part of their personal lives, and recognizing in them an essential part of the message they were to give to the world (Robinson, 1965: 290). White was residing in Australia at the time and provided counsel through a letter delivered at the General Conference session reaffirming that the relationship between the third angel's message and the medical missionary work was to be "as the right arm is to the body," but significantly, she added "the right arm is not to become the whole body" (MM: 312). Furthermore, she strongly emphasized, as she had done on several prior occasions, that a close relationship and co-operation between the ministry and the medical-missionary work must be protected and maintained at all costs. White was unequivocal in her comments, declaring that the "Lord's people are to be one. There is to be no separation in His work. . . . Satan will invent every possible scheme to separate those whom God is seeking to make one" (CH: 517).

History records that the internal struggles and tensions in Adventism concerning the separation between gospel ministers and medical missionary workers continues to reverberate throughout Adventism today. These issues require further exploration as do the principles of Dr. J. H. Kellogg's health reforms, his relationship with and understanding of Ellen White, and the ongoing nature of contemporary institutionalized health care in Seventh-day Adventism.

3

Dr. J. H. Kellogg and Biological Living— the Gospel of Health Reform

IN *LIGHT BEARERS TO the Remnant*, Richard Schwarz argues that very few individuals played a more dominant role in the development of the Seventh-day Adventist church from 1876 to 1904 than Dr. Kellogg. A series of articles published in *Spectrum* in 1990 provides a insight into the diverse and multiple roles that he pursued during his tenure as a Seventh-day Adventist, and in particular his ability to transcend sectarian boundaries and connect with civil society in ways that no Adventist before or since has been able to accommodate.

For more than three decades, Kellogg played a central role in the Seventh-day Adventist church, and no one was as meticulously identified as he was with Adventist teachings on healthful living and the rapidly developing Adventist health care institutions. Few less could match his enthusiasm for ministering to the unemployed, homeless, orphans or the captives of liquor. Kellogg helped meld Adventist education policy, organization of the church's first medical school, and the building the Battle Creek Sanitarium into an institution with both a domestic and international reputation (*Spectrum*, Vol 20, No 3: 46). His facile pen, abundant energy, persistent voice, and creative imagination had made him by 1900 the best-known Seventh-day Adventist among the general public in the USA (Schwarz, 1979: 282).

Kellogg was much more than a cereal maker; however, he was an Adventist giant. Surgeon, inventor, dietician, editor, lecturer, preacher, physician, religious leader and author were some of the titles that the capable doctor assumed. For several years, he directed the International Medical Missionary and Benevolent Association, which employed more workers than the General Conference of SDAs. He organized the denomination's first medical school, with its Chicago branch eventually evolving into the downtown campus of the University of Illinois School of Medicine. 1907, the year Kellogg was disfellowshipped from the Battle Creek Seventh-day Adventist church, witnessed almost 4,000 patients admitted to the Sanitarium (*Spectrum*, Vol 20, No 4: 37).

Kellogg's incessant exploration for more healthful foods helped spawn the prepared breakfast food industry. Furthermore, his inventiveness provided vegetarians with the earliest meat analogs, and interestingly, led Adventists to be known in some quarters as 'peanut eaters.' He was an active member of the General Conference Committee of Seventh-day Adventists, but also found both time and energy to serve on the Michigan State Board of Health and as an adviser to the Women's Christian Temperance Union (*Spectrum*, Vol 20, No 3: 46). He had a unique capacity to combine denominational leadership with managerial responsibilities in a number of organizations and institutions in society, often acting as an 'interface' between his church and society.

Indeed, for more than 50 years Kellogg was a visible entity in American public life (**Spectrum**, Vol 20, No 4: 37). His early contacts with leading European physicians such as Mortimer Granville in London, Pietre-Sante in Paris, and Billroth in Vienna mentored an engaging disposition that led Kellogg to "move freely among captains of industry, government leaders and national and international figures" (*Spectrum*, Vol 20, No 3: 46).

Kellogg passionately cultivated and accepted opportunities to spread Adventist health ideals and reforms in lecture halls as diverse as, Salt Lake City's Mormon Tabernacle (where he addressed 7,000 at the request of Mormon church President William Woodruff in 1898), big city Y.M.C.A's, university campuses and Toledo's municipal park where he was guest of the city's reform mayor, 'Golden Rule' Jones (*Spectrum*, Vol 20, No 3: 46, 47).

The well-known Battle Creek Sanitarium, which Kellogg directed for 67 years, became a favorite retreat of many prominent people in American society. The admission records included a list of celebrities, and business tycoons, such as, John D. Rockefeller, Montgomery Ward, J.C Penny, Alfred

Dupont, and S.S Kresge. The Sanitarium also entertained individuals such as Wall Street genius C. W. Barron, perennial presidential candidate William Jennings Bryan, and conservationist Gifford Pinchot. In 1938, a local newspaper indicated Edgar Welch, the renowned grape juice producer, had visited the 'San' 32 times (*Spectrum*, Vol 20, No 4: 37). Also known to frequent the institution was textile manufacturer Joseph Canon and U.S. Treasurer W. A. Julian who visited the Sanitarium 22 times each (*Spectrum*, Vol 20, No 3: 47). Other 'house-hold' names like Eddie Cantor, Lowell Thomas and the travelers Amundsen, and Richard Halliburton, flocked to the Sanitarium, along with many politicians who enjoyed the establishment's provisions. The "100,000th registered patient was former president William Howard Taft" (*Spectrum*, Vol 20, No 3: 47).

Kellogg's passion for professional contact and dialog with fellow doctors and scientists never diminished. He exchanged visits with the Mayo brothers and the year of the infamous Amadon-Bourdeau interview in 1907 he spent many days observing Pavlov's experiments in St. Petersburg (*Spectrum*, Vol 20, No 3: 47). Kellogg would later bring Pavlov's protégé from Russia to conduct research at Battle Creek. At the personal invitation of the founding editor of the *American Journal of Physical Anthropology*, Kellogg served as one of the journal's early associate editor's.

Prior to the turn of the century, and while still involved in Adventist leadership, Kellogg simultaneously worked alongside Jane Addams, in establishing settlement houses in Chicago, a movement which contributed to the "emergence of the professions of urban planning and social work in America" (*Spectrum*, Vol 20, No 4: 37). Arguably, Kellogg's greatest impact on America emanated from his passion for inculcating healthful living. His publications on sex, such as *Plain Facts About Sexual Life* (in print for 40 years), were among the best sellers of the late nineteenth century in America, and estimates suggest that his fifty books sold over one million copies.

Other complimentary titles bestowed on Kellogg include "the health educator *par excellence*" (Schwarz, 1964: 191), and one of the most influential health educators who ever lived (Schaefer, 1977: 191), as well as deserving of the Nobel Prize for his voluminous writings (Schwarz, 1964: 236). Despite his notable inconsistencies, Kellogg was highly influential, and his ideas, research, and writings influenced not only the Seventh-day Adventist church but the health habits of the United States citizens and the world beyond. Following his death on December 14, 1943, a number of tributes were received from people from all walks of life. Secretary of the US Navy, Frank Knox perhaps summarized best the thoughts of many when stating, "the sudden passing of Dr. Kellogg robs the country of one of its greatest individualists and leaders in medicine. His contribution to national health and well-being was very great and will long be remembered" (Schwarz, 2006: 227).

Thus said, Kellogg remained a controversial character throughout his life and individuals tended to hold polarizing views of the man—they either adored or loathed him. Richard Willis, author of *The Kellogg Imperative* (2003: 11) states that many individuals came to regard Kellogg as both egotistical and bombastic in his style, still friend and foe alike could not ignore or disregard his passionate enthusiasm for his vocation as a medical practitioner, reformer, and health writer, and his inventive genius in health foods and medical equipment. Kellogg was also known to have a sensitive disposition and as such, he disliked criticism and suffered intense periods of depression.

In the contemporary world of Seventh-day Adventism, Kellogg's legacy remains somewhat disputed and continues to polarize discussion resulting in his overall contribution to health reform being diminished and marginalized due to, in particular, his pantheistic views expressed in *The Living Temple* and his eventual expulsion from the SDA church in November, 1907. It would appear that Kellogg's theological aberrations and membership termination from the SDA church have been perceived as a far more serious concern than his health reform advocacy principles were deemed beneficial. His ongoing battles with church administrators and leadership including Ellen White have certainly cast a shadow over the many profound contributions made to health reform. Richard Schwarz, whose extensive research on Kellogg cites a Shakespearian quote when assessing the perception of most Seventh-day Adventists to the health reformers contribution to American society declaring that the "evil that men do lives after them, the good is oft interred with their bones." Therefore, to the majority of Adventists, Schwarz insists, Kellogg remains a dishonorable figure connected with the golden days of the Battle Creek Sanitarium and the early development of 'health foods.' For others, his organizational controversies and theological aberrations have left a tarnished memory and an individual best forgotten. Today, Kellogg's immense efforts to initiate Seventh-day Adventists on a wide-ranging program for alleviating many of American society's social ills remains somewhat unnoticed (Schwarz, 1969: 15). This scenario resonates with the old adage, "throwing the baby out with the bath water." Clearly, these issues require further analysis.

If White provided the visionary experiences supporting health reform, it was Kellogg, more than any other individual in SDA history who implemented the policies and "acted on effecting her inspirational ideas" (Wolfgramm, 1983: 101). Dedication to social welfare was evident through Kellogg's service to the poor, alcoholics, the orphaned and unemployed. He dreamed of the day when Adventism would shed its sectarian image and its adherents would become true medical missionaries or 'Good Samaritans' to the world. He was the social conscience of Seventh-day Adventism for his time (Schwarz and Greenleaf, 1995: 264). During his connection with Adventism, Kellogg achieved more than any other individual in bringing Seventh-day Adventism before the world (SDAE, 1996, vol. 10: 851–853). Numbers insists that from the time of his appointment in 1876 as superintendent of the Western Health Reform Institute, Kellogg had begun to eclipse Ellen White as the church's leading health authority (2008: 230). In many respects, it was Kellogg's aspirations to de-sectarianize Adventism that placed his tenure within the movement in jeopardy.

The Early Years

John Harvey Kellogg, one of sixteen children was born in 1852 in Livingston Country, Michigan, to Mary and John Preston Kellogg, both devout and committed Seventh-day Adventists. As a child, Kellogg moved with his family, first to Jackson, Michigan, and shortly afterwards to Battle Creek, Michigan, where his father commenced a broom factory business venture. Years later J. H. Kellogg and his younger brother William 'Will' Keith Kellogg both put Battle Creek on the map through their industrious work. *The Detroit Free Press* described the brothers as "teamed to bring the world to Michigan and take Michigan to the world" though they could not have had an inkling that this would eventuate when they first arrived in Battle Creek (DFP. 1964: 4B, cited in Willis, 2003: 11, 12).

John's father was prominent among the early Battle Creek Adventists, and his older half-brother, Merritt Kellogg, assisted J. N. Loughborough in opening up Adventist work in California following the Civil War (Dittes, 2013:15). Kellogg's parents were both very active in supporting the Adventist cause and an obituary following his father's death stated that J. P. Kellogg joined the Adventist church in 1852, the same year that John Harvey Kellogg was born, and remained an active member of the Advent movement until his death in 1881, aged 74 years. His first employment opportunity involved organizing and managing tent operations during 1856 in Michigan. He was also part of a three-man Review and Herald publishing committee; one of the Review and Herald publishing association 'corporatores' which was organized in 1861 and one of nine individuals to add their signature to the Western Health Reform Institute articles of incorporation in 1867, and a major subscriber to capital stock (Dittes, 2013: 15). White described Kellogg's mother following her death as a "noble women, true as steel to principle, and I always highly respected her and loved her as a sincere devoted servant of Jesus Christ, as a tried friend, as one whom you knew was reliable under all and every circumstance" (EGW to JHK, Oct. 2, 1893, EGW Estate).

The young J. H. Kellogg displayed his industrious skills at an early age working in his father's broom shop and small store in Battle Creek earning $6 a week in wages. A combination of ill health and minimal emphasis on education among Seventh-day Adventists at the time delayed John Harvey from regular attendance at school until he was nine years of age. He quickly made up for lost time, however, and from the money he earned in the family broom shop, he bought a four-volume set of Farr's Ancient History, and soon had a personal library on botany, shorthand, astronomy, German, and grammar. He also owned a dictionary, and learned to play the violin, piano and organ. (Dittes, 2013: 15, 16).

In 1864, James White visited the Kellogg home and commented on the constructive reports that he had heard concerning John's mental abilities (Schwarz, 2006: 20). Such was the positive impression made that James White invited the 12-year-old to learn the printing trade at the Review and Herald, which White, himself supervised as president of the Seventh-day Adventist Publishing Association (Schwarz, 2006: 20). During the next four years the young Kellogg's progress was rapidly advancing from clean-up, and errand boy to typesetter, proof-reader, and lastly, editorial consultant (Dittes, 2013: 16). Schwarz's analysis is perceptive when declaring that Kellogg's years at the Review and Herald proved immensely significant than he could possibly have realized on that spring day in 1864, for here he received his "first full exposure to the health principles he spent his life in promoting" (2006: 20).

Kellogg originally desired to be a teacher and he maintained a deep interest in chemistry. The influence of family and friends and in particular James and Ellen White was pivotal in mapping out the future vocational trajectory that Kellogg would eventually pursue. They recognized the immense potential in the young lad and persuaded him to take up a career in medicine and provided financial assistance to do so. Kellogg reluctantly agreed with the proposal and first attended Dr Russell Trall's Hygio-Therapeutic College in 1872. His reluctance stemmed from the fact that initially he had no desire or intention of following a medical career; instead, he wanted to become a health educator. History records that he achieved both anyway!

Kellogg graduated with an MD from the six month course; however, he was somewhat disappointed by the whole experience. As such, he opted to make up for the former study program by pursuing further medical studies at the University of Michigan at Ann Arbor and later graduated with a regular MD from the highly prestigious Bellevue Hospital Medical School in New York, considered at that time to be the most advanced medical training institution in the nation (Willis, 2003: 12). It was during this time that Kellogg's editorial writing skills were employed when he became key editorial assistant on *The Health Reformer* at 21 years of age, and within 12 months, Kellogg became editor of the publication.

Such was the measure of the young man's potential that he was invited at just 24 years of age to take over the Western Health Reform Institute in 1876. Kellogg reluctantly agreed when informed that Ellen White supported the appointment, albeit on the understanding that the term of service would be for one year only. Kellogg renamed both the institution and the journal. Indicating his early commitment to an optimistic concept of health, he renamed the institute the 'Battle Creek Sanitarium,' and in the process added the new word 'Sanitarium'—conveying the idea of life and health as opposed to 'Sanitorium', a place for the sick—to the English dictionary. The title of the journal was changed to *Good Health*. Commenting on the change of title in one of his editorials, Kellogg wrote, "If we do not in this journal actually supply the precious boon [good health] itself, we hope to tell the way to find it, and once gained, hope to teach our patrons how to keep it" (Kellogg: 1879: 20). Little did Kellogg realize at the time that he would occupy the same position until his death sixty-seven years later (Schwarz, 1979: 116).

Kellogg's influences as a health reformer, researcher, writer, inventor, surgeon etc, were many and varied. As would be expected, not all Kellogg's ideals and concepts have maintained their veracity through time, however, the scope, breadth and depth of his endeavors were immense, so much so that much of what is now accepted as reliable theory and practice concerning health promotion is anticipated in Kellogg's writings. Clearly, he was not an average individual. While he was a product of his times, his contributions often far exceeded the ability of others to resonate with his thoughts, ideals and processes. He was birthed into a utopia-seeking age, which exerted considerable influence on both his health reform ideals and medical practice. While speaking of White's contribution to health reform, Kellogg also looked for, and found, what he believed was a harmonious and systematic body of hygienic truths, free from patent errors, and entirely consistent with the Bible and the basic principles of the Christian religion (Kellogg, 1890: iii). His well of knowledge ran deep and his emphasis on 'biological living' was central to his health reform schema and it is to that reform agenda that we now direct our attention.

Biological Living—An Integrated Perspective

Anne Riley Hale, an anti-medical propagandist in the 1920s defined the indispensable credo of health reform as the belief that "the Kingdom of Health, like the Kingdom of Heaven, is within you" and can be achieved by hygienic righteousness (Whorton, 1982: 4). Many health reformers of the day would have concurred with Hale's analysis. Disease theory was in its infancy at the time but would soon be enveloped by a burgeoning health reform movement. The main approach to health fostered in the new American colony was based on the religious ideals of the immigrants who sought refuge from the persecuting European powers (Willis, 2003: 15). Bryan Ball (1981) has documented the wide-ranging impact that the health teachings of the Puritan immigrants contributed, including the wholistic concept of humanity, vegetarianism, and temperance in eating and drinking. Health reform, therefore, merged forces with Enlightenment processes and secular scientism resulting in a movement characterized by its highly moralized pronouncements.

In touch with the reality of the world enveloping him, Kellogg wrote that it is "high time that those who are seeking to reform the world should begin to preach the gospel of health" (1893: v). As noted previously, during the early to mid-nineteenth century in America, individuals increasingly came to believe that they could no longer accept the notion that humanity was too depraved to play any part or role in their own salvation. Revivalism provided both the rationale and the means for Americans, acting together in good will to join in a mass effort to seek and secure their own salvation (McLoughlin, 1974: 142). While this new style of evangelical revivalism was not universally accepted and caused some division and resentment it did provide a forum for a growing awareness of the ability of the individual to diversify and pursue all manner of reforms, including health (Ferret, 2008: 32). Hancock declares that it was "a utopian society," and furthermore, respectable utopian thinking provides not only a beacon to light our way for the future, and a goal to strive to achieve; but it also tells us "what we would like the world to be, as opposed to what we think it will be like" (1992: 22).

Morality and health reform often proceeded 'hand-in-hand,' for a developing view of high morality was a characteristic of the age. The increasingly robust emphasis on spiritual perfection stressed in the religious revivals of the time and which dominated the age was soon translated into the necessity for physical perfection (Willis, 2003: 16). Reid argues that Sylvester Graham's (1974–1851) most significant contribution to the health reform movement was combining the issues of health and morality into a single package, which in turn, provided the needed motivation to inspire action (1982: 36). Kellogg, himself a religious person, deemed health to be a core part of Christian living and that humanity was in dire need of restoration to God's ideals (Willis, 2003: 9). Referring to this restoration principle, he would write:

> The guidance of infinite wisdom is as much needed in the discerning between truth and error as in the evolution of new truths. Novelty is by no means a distinguishing characteristic of true principles, and the principle holds good as regards the truths of hygienic reform, as well as those of other reformatory movements. The greatest and most important reformatory movements of modern times have not been those which presented new facts and principles but those which revived truths and principles long forgotten, and by which have led the way back to the paths trodden by men of by-gone ages, before the world had wandered so far from physical and moral rectitude. (1890: iv)

Thus, for Kellogg, health reform was not an addition to life that could be adopted based on one's duty; no, it was to be established as a *way of life*. He continues by declaring that if individuals undertake to go about this thing in a willing way, God will enlighten their minds, and he will lead them into correct ways. "I think," he reasoned, "that people years ago tried to live out health reform from a sense of duty, and just as soon as they would begin to backslide a little, they would abandon it altogether" (1897 [1]: 135).

Horace Mann, a prominent educational reformer at the time also articulated the developing merger between the physical and the spiritual dimensions when suggesting that in all things, humanity should obey the physical laws of god, for they would no more "suffer physical pain, than they would suffer remorse, or moral pain, if in all they would obey the moral laws of God (Reid, 1982: 25). Willis (2003: 16) notes that this merging of the spiritual and the physical is continually expressed in the writings of nineteenth-century health reformers and has persisted well into the following centuries, citing Christian Science as a prime example.

Schwarz observes that it was during his course as a medical student at Bellevue Hospital Medical School in New York, that Kellogg outlined in the journal *Health Reformer* the basic principles of healthful living that he would continue to promote throughout his life. The author elaborates further declaring that the essence of his system, for which he eventually coined the phrase 'biological living,' was, in reality, preventative medicine at its very best for it had as its goal the desire help people stay well, rather than to just recover from illness (2006: 40).

Kellogg insisted that *biological living* was, in fact, an integrated system replete with several components including proper diet, adequate water, hydropathic treatments (hot and cold baths, packs, fomentations etc.), exercise, correct posture and appropriate dress, adequate rest, and exposure to enough sunlight (Schwarz, 2006: 57). Kellogg's influence, however, was distinctive in that he sought to combine preventative health measures with emerging scientific evidence to support his reforms. The doctor, himself, was often at the forefront of these trial endeavors, always seeking to discover a better solution in alleviating the ills of humankind. He was often ridiculed of 'making mountains out of molehills' or being a fanatic due to his enthusiastic promotion of a particular aspect of a healthful lifestyle.

Richard Schwarz's biography titled, *John Harvey Kellogg: Pioneering Health Reformer*, elaborates in depth the major components that formed the basis of Kellogg's health reform agenda, and the following is a condensation of those features. Kellogg maintained that obedience to the natural laws of health was essential for the maintenance of moral, mental and physical health, and as such became a personal, moral duty. His views were not unique in relation to many other contemporary reformers, who, like Kellogg, suggested that abstinence from tea, coffee, alcohol, and tobacco would prolong both health and longevity. Kellogg also insisted that in the event of illness, simple, and as far as possible, natural remedies remain the safest and most productive form of treatment.

A proper diet was at the core of health maintenance, and no food suffered a more sustained attack from Kellogg than meat products. Such was his conviction, and contrary to public opinion, the doctor "believed that eating meat was a major precipitating factor in diseases of the circulatory system and the kidneys, that it encouraged high blood pressure and anemia, and that it was probably largely responsible for such diseases as cancer, diabetes, and apoplexy." He also warned that a meat diet would likely contribute to more complaints including headaches, constipation and would delay recovery from skin disorders, tuberculosis, and mental disorders. Initially milk, eggs and cheese did not escape Kellogg's culinary suspicion; however, he eventually modified his views acknowledging that fresh cheese was more preferable than meat as a source of protein and in 1917 stated that milk was "the choicest product of nature's laboratory." Kellogg remained unmoved concerning his dislike for eggs as suitable for human consumption, although he did slightly acquiesce suggesting that eggs may be helpful to supplement a diet lacking in vitamins, proteins, lime and iron, and as long as the eggs were both fresh and well cooked.

Sweet foods never fared well with Kellogg, particularly cane sugar, as it was understood to interfere with proper digestion and the excessive use of sweets deemed more dangerous to the diet than some meat products. Whilst the energetic doctor did not favor the total elimination of sugar from the diet he believed that "sweet-toothed" Americans, with their love of candy and sweet desserts needed to bring their desires under rigid control. Kellogg insisted that natural sweets, such as dates, honey and raisins should be utilized whenever possible. Salt was placed in the same undesirable category as sugar, and if used at all it should be very sparingly. Kellogg was satisfied that natural foods contained enough salt to provide for normal human body requirements.

Condiments, as was the case with most contemporary health reformers, were quickly added to 'banned list.' Mustard, cinnamon, ginger, pepper and other spices, along with pickles, were destined to be eliminated from consumption on the basis that condiments stimulated the stomach's activity while simultaneously inhibiting the necessary secretion of gastric juices. Kellogg's 'rule of thumb' was that if foods which were 'hot' when they were actually cold were unfit for consumption.

Vegetarianism was an attractive alternative for Kellogg, although for many years he declined to introduce any vegetables, other than legumes, to his restrictive dietary habits. He initially determined that any vegetables that grew under the ground did not receive sunlight, therefore, they were deficient, although again, as health reforms became aligned with a more progressive and expanding scientific understanding, changes were adopted as appropriate. In later years, he reversed his views concerning vegetables that grow underground and actively promoted potatoes, "convinced that the higher alkali content of root vegetables made them better food than most grains." A similar scenario existed regarding the eating of raw vegetables. Originally, the doctor saw little, if any, benefit in consuming raw vegetables, but later modified his views and suggested that a little raw food each day is good for the constitution.

Fruit maintained a special place in Kellogg's recommended diet. He believed that a variety of fruits should occupy central place on American household dining tables, as fruit was not a luxury but a necessity. Ripened fruits were considered the most nutritious and easily digested of all the food types available, and Kellogg was often observed handing a variety of fruits to both his associates and patients. Nuts fared equally as well as fruit and the doctor considered that nuts were 'pound for pound' the most nutritious food.

Excessive eating by the general populace also frustrated Kellogg for he was convinced that overeating caused permanent damage to the digestive organs, and obesity placed enormous strain on the circulatory system, kidneys and liver and made them vulnerable to chronic disorders. The challenge for overweight people, Kellogg insisted, was to halve their daily calorie intake from their present intake and in the process include bulky, laxative foods such as fresh green vegetables. It almost goes without saying; sweets of all kinds were not to be tolerated. When a regular exercise program, and sweat baths were included, the doctor believed restoration of normal weight and health would follow.

For a number of years Kellogg advocated limiting food consumption to two meals per day with at least six hours between them. For those reluctant to dispose of a third daily meal, Kellogg's response was to institute the heaviest meal at midday and the lightest meal in the evening as an overfull and extended stomach interfered with a restful sleep (Schwarz, 2006: 40–50).

Biological Living—Kellogg's Theology

Thomas A. Edison (1847–1931), a contemporary of Kellogg insightfully wrote that the "doctor of the future will give no medication, but will interest his patients in the care of the human frame, in diet, and in the cause and prevention of disease" (Werbach, 1986: 179). While Edison may not have had Dr. J. H. Kellogg specifically in mind, the aptness of his description to Kellogg's biological living is quite remarkable (Willis, 2003: 40).

In 1898, Kellogg wrote an article titled, "The Greater Gospel," in which he penned the following lines: "We must recognize as a solemn reality that religion includes the body, and that the laws which govern the healthful performance of the bodily functions are as much the laws of God as those of the Decalogue" (1903: 431). Citing the Hebrew's Exodus from Egyptian slavery in the Old Testament, Kellogg elaborates further:

> The gospel of deliverance which Moses taught offered redemption from physical as well as moral degeneracy. In instructing his people in the wilderness, God did not stop at the so-called Decalogue, or moral law, but supplemented it by a code of sanitary regulations which have been the recognized model during all ages since. The sanitary code of Moses included minute instructions about diet, cleanliness, clothing, domestic sanitation, disinfection, and quarantine; and the out-of-door life and constant moving from place to place, the pure diet of manna, and the crystal pure water from the rock afforded the conditions essential for physical regeneration and a return to natural and original simplicity, while the daily instruction in moral principles given by Moses and his associates, was the means of educating a semi-barbarous horde up to a level of godly people. (1903: 431–439)

Kellogg insisted that humankind's supreme obligation to the Creator is to the follow the principles of biological living, declaring that God's desire "for the prosperity of the *health* of man is exactly on an equality with His wish for the prosperity of the *soul* of man." Thus, "when it came to holiness," declares Wilson, Kellogg firmly believed that "purity of body was equally important for salvation as purity of soul, and, indeed, it would be difficult to heal the soul without first healing the body." Of course, Kellogg was not the first to echo the sentiments that health reform precedes theological reforms. Dr. Caleb Jackson, of hydrotherapy fame and director of 'Our home on the Hillside' in Dansville, New York, the same institution that James and Ellen White visited in 1864 seeking treatment, believed that "when it came to saving souls, health reform should take precedence over preaching." In other words, "health reform would replace revivals for the conversion of souls" (Wilson, 2014: 30). Kellogg, in a similar vein was adamant "that the Christian doctor was destined for a role in salvation at least as important—if not so more—than that of a minister of the gospel." The Battle Creek Sanitarium's rationale for existence, in the mind of Kellogg, was "designed to function as a 'gospel agency' to evangelize the world in the principles of 'biological living'" (Wilson, 2014: 50, 51). Those principles were outlined in an 1875 editorial named "The Hygienic Platform."

1. Obedience to the laws of life and health is a moral obligation.

2. Mental, moral, and physical health can only be maintained by the observance of mental, moral, and physical laws.

3. A healthy body is essential to perfect soundness of mind.

4. Physical health promotes morality.

5. Morality, likewise, promotes physical health.

6. In the treatment of disease the simplest and safest remedies are the proper curative agents.

7. Nature is the most efficient physician. (Wilson, 2014: 44)

Dr Clive McCay, formerly professor of nutrition at Cornell University dated the genesis of modern nutritional science around 1900 (Coon, 1993: 11), while Reid notes that in the "1860s even scientists knew little of modern human nutrition, and the public had only folklore for guidance" (1982: 138). If earlier nineteenth-century health reformers had made the initial attempt to base nutrition within a scientific context, it was predominantly Kellogg "who carried the work forward" (Willis, 2003: 44). Horace Powell insists that while Kellogg may have seemed revolutionary to his more conservative colleagues, he actually was restating and implementing basic health ideas, which had been in the minds of men for several centuries (1956: 55).

Kellogg consistently endeavored to merge science and religion into the pragmatics of health reform in a rapidly changing world. In his 1921 publication, *The New Dietetics*, a book described by philosopher Will Durrant as deserving of the Nobel Prize (Schwarz, 1964: 236), Kellogg spoke of his interest and personal efforts in the promotion of scientifically based nutritional and dietetic reforms:

There is perhaps no place in the world where the successive steps of scientific progress in the knowledge of nutrition and dietetics have been watched with greater care and interest than at Battle Creek Sanitarium. For more than forty years this institution has been a great clinical laboratory in which an intensive study of foodstuffs and of their effect upon the human body has been continuously carried on by the writer and his associates. . . . It is not claimed that complete knowledge has yet been attained. . . . the writer desires to ask the readers' consideration of the fact that however widely the ideas and methods herein may differ from those current in popular and professional usage, they cannot be justly looked upon as simply theoretical or experimental, since they are in daily use in a large institution, in the development of which during the last forty-five years they are believed to have been an important factor. However novel the methods presented may seem to some readers, they are by no means new; they are based upon *biological principles* which are as old as the human race and only need a fair trial to demonstrate their value.

While virtually all aspects of Dr. J. H. Kellogg's biological living appear in various forms in the teachings of earlier health reformers along with the writings of White (Schwarz, 2006: 57), it was his attempts to synthesize his Seventh-day Adventist theological views with the escalating scientific and medical discoveries of his time that became his constant struggle. The intellectual life of Kellogg was contextualized by continual doubts fueled in part by scientific inquiry and the advent of Darwinism. Other contributing factors included the challenges associated with religious progress, doctrinal revisions involving original sin and soul immortality, the growing impact of industrialization and commercialism on religious values, fundamentalism verses modernism, and sectarianism verses ecumenism (Carter, 1971). Thus, as Wilson aptly states, "the new theology behind biological living was first and foremost an expression of Kellogg's very real and very personal struggle to reconcile religion with science and medicine" (2014: xiv).

The life and times of Dr. J. H. Kellogg have received serious investigation by both denominational and secular historians with Richard W. Schwarz's biographical publication, *John Harvey Kellogg: Pioneering Health Reformer* published in 2006, a recognized standard. In 2014, Brian C. Wilson, Professor in the Department of Comparative Religion at Western Michigan University published a book titled, *Dr. John Harvey Kellogg and the Religion of Biological Living*, which explores in detail, perhaps for the first time, Kellogg's theological development or "the doctor as theologian" (2014: xiii).

Kellogg's increasing success as an administrator, doctor, surgeon, writer, etc., brought in its wake increased scrutinization from both the medical profession and his church, resulting in essentially a 'tug-of-war' between religious allegiance or scientific respectability. His trial with Calhoun County Medical Board in 1886 which posed a serious threat to his professional reputation was based on what was deemed 'unbecoming of a regular physician,' that is, his promotion of biological living. Whilst eventually exonerated, this episode resulted in Kellogg redoubling his efforts to protect his professional status in the medical field and perhaps provides an insight into his rationale for insisting that the Battle Creek Sanitarium be conducted from a non-denominational or sectarian mission. Wilson suggests that it is "not coincidental that during this period, Dr. Kellogg began to move decisively away from many of the specific dogmas of Seventh-day Adventism and to equip his biological living with a more modernist theological rationale" (Wilson, 2014: 62).

It would appear that from a young age Kellogg harbored a good measure of helpful skepticism, which would remain his constant companion. A story Kellogg was fond of reciting occurred when he was seven or eight years old involving his dismissal from a church Sabbath school class for impertinence. The young inquiring Kellogg had dared to ask his teacher why an all-powerful God would create a bad, instead of a good Devil. The young lad posed the same question to his father on his return home, only to be quickly silenced again. Kellogg was confused as to why his questions elicited no response, but instead, condemnation. "From then on, declares Wilson, "Kellogg would make up his own mind about theological questions" (Wilson, 2014: 64).

The young doctor's skepticism did not abate but only deepened throughout his medical education, and in particular, his exposure to philosophical materialism of the natural sciences seriously influenced his views of religion. Dr Palmer, a natural treatment advocate enjoined Kellogg and his fellow students to consider the human body in "thoroughly materialistic and mechanistic ways." That is, the "human body can be compared to a watch or an engine which have valves, wheels, pistons, cylinders etc.," If these malfunction a mechanic is enlisted "who understands the problem." Likewise, "the doctor is simply the mechanic of the body, and the body simply a machine, and if that was the case, religious meanings of the body" were inconsequential and little use in treating disease. Could it be that Kellogg's medical education "imbibed deeply the idea that religion and medicine" do not mix well? (Wilson, 2014: 65).

A filial relationship existed between Ellen White and J. H. Kellogg (Willis, 2003: 35). In 1899, Kellogg wrote to Ellen White that he had loved and respected her as his own mother.

On one occasion he stated, "I have always entertained the greatest respect and regard for Mrs. White. Aside from my parents, she was the best friend I ever had. She treated me like a son. As a young man I was a member of her family" (1938). In a real sense, White was Kellogg's surrogate mother, often times nurturing him, sometimes rebuking him. Kellogg would sometimes confide in her his guilt as a result of his "inability to take all aspects of his Adventist faith at face value" (Wilson, 2014: 6). On one such occasion, he wrote her, "I have a theoretical faith, but am of such a doubting suspicious nature that I cannot make practical application of it" (Schwarz, 1970: 62, 63).

While doubts continued, Kellogg never deserted his faith, nor did he adopt completely, a materialistic worldview. Wilson elaborates: "The fact he was a doctor—a man of science—made the problem more acute, but instead of abandoning his faith altogether, he spent the rest of his life trying to harmonize science with religion and construct a theology that would allow him to honor both" (2014: 65). This proved to be an unenviable task indeed!

In 1876, shortly after assuming directorship of the Battle Creek Sanitarium, Kellogg felt obligated to reconcile in print some of his Adventist beliefs with the growing materialism of medicine and science. He had already experienced the sting of accusations by fellow Adventists of maintaining "infidel sentiments," but was exonerated by the passing of a resolution at the 1878 General Conference in Battle Creek. In 1879, *Harmony of Science and the Bible* was published by the Review and Herald Publishing Association in Battle Creek, resulting, as far as Kellogg was concerned, in successfully reconciling "three Adventist beliefs with scientific doctrine: bodily resurrection, 'soul sleep' and conditional immortality (Wilson, 2014: 66 70). Interestingly, Kellogg commenced his discussion in his new publication arguing that there would be "no conflict between religion and science if only Christians would not insist on literal readings of Holy Writ and not let their superstitious fear stand in the way of scientific, especially medical, progress" (Wilson, 2014: 66). In the respect, Dr. Kellogg is characteristically an Enlightenment modernist.

Given the pressure of ongoing scientific developments in the 1890s, Kellogg was continually preoccupied about the continual impact of science on religion in general, and his own faith in particular. The two central aspects that troubled Kellogg the most in his quest for reconciliation were "the Adventist's highly anthropomorphic conception of God localized in heaven and the relationship of this remote God with the material cosmos." In light of the contemporary naturalistic assumptions of modern evolutionary theory in biology, geology and cosmology, this presupposed either an 'idle God' of deism or "explained the cosmos in terms of completely mechanistic processes" (Wilson, 2014: 70, 71). Kellogg found himself in a major quandary. In a later recollection in 1897 he states, "I was trying to believe in God and nature. I had two Gods. But I could not go on thus. I could not see how God could be above nature, so I had taken the position that God was not above nature. . . . I believed that nature [was] almost equal with God" (GCDB, Feb. 18, 1897). Kellogg, once again, confided his concerns to White who responded by seeking to help the doctor reject both scientific materialism and deism in favor of anthropomorphic theism:

> Christ and the Father are continually working through the laws of nature. Those who dwell on the laws of matter and the laws of nature, in following their own limited, finite understanding, lose sight of, if they do not deny, the continual and direct agency of God. Many express themselves in a manner which would convey the idea that nature is distinct from the God of nature, having in and of itself its own limits and its own powers wherewith to work. There is with many a marked distinction between natural and supernatural. The natural is ascribed to ordinary causes, unconnected with the interference with God. Vital power is attributed to matter, and nature is made a deity. Matter is supposed to be placed in certain relations, and left to act from fixed laws, with which God himself cannot interfere; that nature is endowed with certain properties and placed subject to laws, and left to itself to obey these laws, and perform the work originally commanded. This is false science; there is nothing in the Word of God to sustain it. God does not annul his laws, but he is continually working through them, using them as his instruments. They are not self-working. (GCDB, February 18, 1897)

White elaborated further on what she regarded as the false science of deifying nature, declaring instead, that God is continuously engaged in nature:

> Nature in her work testifies of the intelligent presence and active agency of a Being who moves in all his works according to his will. It is not by an original power inherent in nature that year by year the earth produces its bounties, and the world keeps up its continual march around the sun. The hand of infinite power is perpetually at work guiding this planet. It is God's power momentarily exercised that keeps it in position in its rotations. The God of heaven is constantly at work. It is by his power that vegetation is caused to flourish, that every leaf appears and every flower blooms. It is not as the result of a mechanism, that, once set in motion, continues its work, that the pulse beats and breath follows breath. In God we live and move and have our being. Every breath, every throb of the heart, is the continual evidence of the power of an ever-present God. (GCDB, February 18, 1897)

Kellogg was initially relieved by the content of White's letter, for he still considered her prophetic counsel divinely inspired at this time. Thus, it was not merely human opinion he was confronted with in White's counsel, but instead, utter truth vouchsafed by God. The doctor experienced intense joy at the realization that empirical science was still subservient to divine revelation. His initial enthusiasm would not last long, however, and soon he felt the need to rework White's characterization of God in the cosmos due to its apparent vagueness, but perhaps more significantly, because he was still very uncomfortable with an anthropomorphic God (Wilson, 2014: 71, 72).

Contemporary critics of Kellogg labelled his theological meanderings pantheism; God and nature are one. Kellogg insisted that "nature is simply a philosophical name for God" (1903: 483). Later, a more precise label was designated declaring his theological position as the doctrine of divine immanence or immanent theism, which argued that God and nature are separate, but nonetheless, God is always present in nature. Regardless of the label given, Kellogg became convinced that his understanding of God as immanent in the world was "the great truth which harmonizes all correct religious views and principles—every truth that is essential to man's salvation harmonizes with one great central truth" (Wilson, 2014: 72).

1897 provided the defining moment for Kellogg's theology of divine immanence to be made public. In an address to the General Conference of Seventh-day Adventists in Lincoln, Nebraska, Kellogg delivered a series of lectures entitled "God in Man." The content of his lectures did not provide new information; however, the radical implications of his theology were quickly noted. "What a wonderful thought," Kellogg declared to his audience, "that this mighty God that keeps the whole universe in order, is in us!" Indeed, for Kellogg, the most notable aspect of God's immanence was that "God actually designs to be the intelligence behind the so-called autonomic functions of the human body—that breath, heartbeat, digestion, muscular contraction, nervous system were all the continual work of God" (GCDB, No.1, Feb. 18, 1987). Kellogg's 'God in man' emphasis soon became 'God is man's servant' theory as noted in his following statement:

> When we look at the fact that man is the masterpiece of God; that when God made him, he pronounced him very good; that after he made everything else—the earth, the world, the animals, everything,—he said to his son, Let us make man in our own image;—when we think of that, that God has taken clay and animated that clay, put into that clay his own self, put himself into it, so he has made in the mass of clay a godlike man, absolutely put divinity in the earth, and has given me a will, and has made himself the servant of that will, we see that God is man's servant. (GCDB, No. 3, Feb. 19, 1987)

Kellogg's radical theological conclusions regarding 'God as the servant of man' led also to the adoption of a radical perfectionism. He was quick to explain to his Adventist audience that if human beings could simply recognize the fact that God dwells in them literally, and if they would cooperate with God in obedience to both physical and moral laws, then they too could achieve the physical and moral perfection in this life that Jesus achieved in his. The rationale for Kellogg was clear, for "the same divinity that was in Christ is in us, and is ever seeking to lead us to the same perfection which we see in Christ. To the attainment of which there can be no hindrance except our individual wills" (GCDB, No. 1, Feb. 18, 1987). While the nature of perfection was a constant Adventist theme at the time (and one which continues into the present), the idea that physical and moral perfection could be achieved on the basis of the indwelling God was new, and furthermore, the implications that Kellogg drew from his perfectionistic views "were now leading him to question, not defend, some key Adventist doctrines" (Wilson, 2014: 76).

Shortly following the Nebraska conference, White opened a letter from Dr. Kellogg, where he outlined the implications of his developing theology regarding biological living. He wrote that those ready for Christ when he comes will be above the power of sin including all diseases, and this condition will be achieved by obedience to truth. He maintained that the sealing of God is both a moral and physical change which takes place in the individual as a result of adhering to truth and which shows in their countenance that it is, indeed, the seal of God, and furthermore, the mark of the beast is the mark of the work of the beast in the heart that changes the body as well as the character and also shows in one's countenance (Schwarz, 1972: 23–29). The implications were quite obvious, "Satan's seal was simply the physical ugliness of an unhealthy body, whereas the seal that God places on human beings as an outward mark of their worthiness for salvation is physical health, if not physical beauty" (Wilson, 2014: 76). These themes, Kellogg insisted, should be the focal point of Seventh-day Adventist theology, for "it seems to me" he would write, "our people have been wrong in regarding Sunday observance as the sole mark of the beast. . . . The mark of the beast . . . is simply the change in character and body that comes from the surrender of the will to Satan" (Schwarz, 1972: 24). The true seal of the remnant people, Kellogg argued, was not to be specifically associated with Sabbath observance or worship as an identifying mark of the elect, rather, it the seal involved the "physical and moral perfection that comes from biological living" (Wilson, 2014: 76).

While Kellogg had declared that the quest for physical perfection is the sign of the millennial seal among the remnant in his presentation, "God in Man," delivered during the 1897 General Conference, he went one step further in another lecture, "The Physical Basis of Faith." On this occasion, his theology became more radicalized when he declared that physical perfection provided the potential for the elect to escape death. "The only thing necessary for a man to live forever is an abundance of life. If we had it all the time we might live forever." How is this abundant life achieved? Through dietary practice. That is, death results primarily through the consumption of flesh foods, whereas indefinite life is only achievable through a vegetarian diet. Thus, if "only human beings would restrict themselves to a vegetarian diet, then their lives would never end" (Wilson, 2014: 79).

In another presentation in 1901, Kellogg pushed his 'indefinite life' motif further stating that because Jesus never sinned, either physiologically or morally, he would have lived forever if men had not ended his life. The implications of these concepts on Atonement theology, in particular, become clearly evident. The true meaning of Christ's atonement was not to be associated with his substitutionary death at Calvary, nor anything to do with his heavenly sanctuary ministry, but rather, his "exemplary life, demonstrating to mankind that spiritual and physical perfection was possible" and, as such, "indefinite life, could be striven for by people on earth" (Wilson, 2014: 79). If the atonement was based on Christ's exemplary moral and physiological life alone, then what did this mean for the Adventist sanctuary doctrine? In April 1901, Kellogg provided his answer, and in doing so took aim at Adventism's literalist interpretation of Scripture:

> Now, we have the doctrine of the Sanctuary. Many people have never really believed that, because it was so architectural. . . . Now the belief is almost entirely a material one. One sees three or four rooms set apart in Heaven or somewhere, and Christ walking back and forth from one room to another. This has been a perfectly terrible thing to believe. Two years ago it dawned upon me, when reading the 10th of Hebrews, that the Body was the Sanctuary. . . . And that is the whole message, the restoration of the Kingdom, Christ taking possession again, and the cleansing of the sanctuary—our bodies—so that Christ can work in us. . . . Now that doctrine is so simple and so beautiful that when I go out into the world with that doctrine, and tell them that man is upon such a different level—instead of being simply a clod of clay that dies and rots and goes down into the earth, he is the temple of the living God, he is the true tabernacle of God. (cited in Wilson, 2014: 80)

The ramifications of Kellogg's divine immanence theology could be felt throughout the Adventist movement, for the implications were so broad that they impacted virtually every tenet of the SDA faith including doctrines such as, the nature of sin, the seal of God, Sabbath observance, death and resurrection, atonement, perfection, and heavenly sanctuary, to mention a few. For Kellogg, the sanctuary was not in heaven, rather, it was on earth; the human body constituting the living temple of God.

Kellogg was convinced that the theology of divine immanence provided the missing link in Adventist theology by achieving the amalgamation of doctrinal integrity with scientific enquiry. Referring to this success, he wrote:

> The time has come when our principles are at a point where we can meet any kind of opposition, and so can talk all our different doctrines, the diet question, the meat question, the dress question, they have all reached a point where they are in perfect harmony and have a scientific foundation that the world will recognize, and

our religious faith, our theological doctrines are all in harmony with it so that the time has come when the truth can go out into the world with a harmonious simplicity that intelligent people all over the world can recognize. (cited in Wilson, 2014: 80, 81)

The Living Temple published in 1903 contained little that Kellogg had not previously advocated during the previous decade, however, the book did present the author's theology of biological living in its most complete form. Statements in the first chapter provide the context for the remainder of the book. "God is the explanation of nature—not a God outside nature, but in nature, manifesting himself through and in all objects, movements, and various phenomena of the universe" (Kellogg, 1903: 28). This immanence of God was so pervasive that in nature, every living thing, from the minute microbe and cell to leaf and flowers were all continually being created by the indwelling power of God. Furthermore,

> There is present in the tree a power which creates and maintains it, a tree-maker in the tree, a flower-maker in the flower—a divine architect who understands every law of proportion, an infinite artist who possesses a limitless power of expression in color and form; there is, in all the world about us, an infinite, divine, though visible Presence, to which the unenlightened may be blind, but which is ever declaring itself by its ceaseless beneficent activity. (Kellogg, 1903: 29)

The author continues declaring that just like the trees and plants, "God dwells in man," in fact "He is the life of man," and in the very process of digestion, or "transfiguration" as Kellogg suggested, humans are actually ingesting the very power of God (Kellogg, 1903: 36). In the same book, Kellogg also reiterated his belief that God was the servant of man inhabiting both believer and unbeliever alike and providing divine power for the actions of both. Again, the implications become evident, in that, "all that was necessary for human perfection, physical *and* spiritual, was simply to choose to live in harmony with God was, of course, biological living, which, since God lived in us, could be practiced by either saint or sinner" (Wilson, 2014: 87).

Wilson discusses the many sources that possibly influenced Kellogg's pantheistic views in his chapter *The Living Temple*, including tensions from within Adventism regarding the ongoing trinitarianism debate, but also a number of other significant factors:

The important conclusion . . . is that although Kellogg would remain sectarian in his emphasis on biological living, the immanent theology behind it actually brought him closer to the liberal theological mainstream of America. Kellogg never called himself a modernist, but both his theology and his nondenominational ecclesiology bore all the modernist hall marks. . . . Driven by his desire to desire to reconcile science with religion, Kellogg naturally gravitated in this direction, and, indeed, he always claimed that his study of biology forced him to accept the truth of divine immanence. (2014: 101)

In 1906, Kellogg declared that "the evidences that this world's history is drawing to a close are so many and so conclusive that no room is left to doubt or question the meaning of the prophetic vision which has stood as a warning to the world during so many generations." Kellogg continues arguing that "the only hope for the saving of even a few from the approaching ruin is through intelligent, consistent medical work, based upon the foundation of a return to natural, simple habits of life, the recognition of the natural order which God established in Eden as the divine order" (Kellogg, 1906: 129–133).

As previously noted, Kellogg maintained that God's remnant believers would not be saved on the basis of doctrinal adherence, be it Sabbath observance or whatever, but instead, only through the practice of biological living within an apocalyptic context. The nature or character of the coming apocalypse was the decisive issue. That is, would the coming calamity be a result of supernatural intervention as depicted in the book of Revelation or because of more naturalistic causes? Kellogg "opted for the latter" with 'race degeneration' and eugenics becoming his preferred 'apocalyptic narrative" (Wilson, 2014: 137).

It is critical that Kellogg's 'race degeneration' ideals be socio-historically located so as to avoid him being designated a 'racist' when measured against current time and sensibilities. Ideas concerning race degeneration and decreasing longevity did not originate with Kellogg, for they were prominent in the ranks of other antebellum Christian physiologists such as Graham, Alcott and Blackwell (Engs, 2000: 69–74). Human hereditary processes and their association with physical anthropology was a developing field of study in the late nineteenth and early twentieth century and there were three widespread beliefs held. The first involved the inheritability of certain types of disease (tuberculosis, gout, cancer, heart disease). Certain negative character traits that led to disease comprised the second belief (e.g. excessive sexual desire or intemperance). The third belief involved the related concept of heritability of acquired character-istics, called Larmarckianism, after the early nineteenth-century French naturalist, Jean-Baptiste Lamarch (Wilson, 2014: 138). Larmarckianism provided "a mechanism by which the health and moral character of chil-dren were the result of individual actions of the parents, so that if a parent either improved or impaired him—or—herself through virtuous or im-moral practices, the child would consequently experience better or worse character and health" (Wilson, 2014: 138).

These degenerative processes whilst evident were not a cause for pessi-mism. The "good news was that the degenerative process could be stopped if only men and women would follow the laws of health . . . the doleful effects of race degeneration going all the way back to the fall could be completely reversed after a few generations" (Wilson, 2014: 139). Essentially, biological living "could upgrade the individual" (Willis, 2003: 86). Indeed, this was a most thrilling prospect to William Alcott whose unrestrained pen would write: "Whose heart does not beat high at the bare possibility of becoming the progenitor of the world, as it were, of pure, healthy, and greatly elevated beings—a race worthy of emerging from the fall—and estamping on it a species of immortality" (Engs, 2000: 67, 74).

Kellogg imbibed these ideas of human heredity as propounded by the Christian physiologists declaring that "the effects of . . . wholesale poison-ing are apparent in every civilized land in the obvious degeneracy which is taking place" (cited in Wilson, 2014: 141). The key to the Christian physi-ologist's understanding of hereditary was again highlighted under the ban-ner of Larmarckianism:

> The physician whose eyes have been enlightened sees in much of the conduct of human beings which is charged to individual depravity, in the nervousness, wrongheadedness, weakness of will, and over mastering propensities, the hereditary results of whiskey drinking, tobacco smoking, selfindulgent fathers; or tea drinking, corset wearing, fashion enslaved mothers. (cited in Wilson, 2014: 139)

Dietary taboos such as alcohol, tobacco, caffeine, and the consump-tion of flesh foods along with constricting clothing, were considered 'race poisons' and their detrimental impact was not restricted to those who consumed them, but to the individuals offspring also. Larmarckianism was "just too important for the plausibility of biologic living for it to be abandoned" by Kellogg. (Wilson, 2014: 140).

Another important factor was that Kellogg came to fear that his country was experiencing a "rapid acceleration of race degeneration." While the increasing availability of race poisons such as alcohol, tobacco and bad diet contributed to race degeneration, improvements in public health and sanitation was particularly singled out for special attention because it "led to a situation where the weak survived and reproduced, thus diminishing the constitutional vigor of the race." (Wilson, 2014: 142).

Perhaps one of the more sensational theories being discussed in the early 1900s was that the "Anglo-Saxon race was in danger of being weakened by intermarriage with 'lesser races' and was thus in danger of losing the energy and will to fulfil its global civilizing and Christianizing mission." (Wilson, 2014: 143). Kellogg agreed and suggested that to avoid race suicide the white race must adopt biologic living thus producing more and healthier children, and avoid mixed marriages if possible. As much as he admired certain individuals within the black American race, Kellogg's overall opinion of the potential for the African American race was poor: "The intellectual inferiority of the negro male to the European male is universally acknowledged" was penned in 1902 (1902: 193). In 1908, he concurred with a paper he reported on that contended that "the causes of the degeneration of the negro were clearly the outgrowth of immorality, and . . . that no degree of education and no mere sanitary or social measures could possibly save the negro from degeneracy and extinction" (1908: 58). God may have created humankind as one, but nature thought otherwise, he believed. Furthermore, the "subsequent exposure to climatic extremes had created subspecies, which, though all equally worthy in the sight of God, were nevertheless biologically incompatible and intellectually unequal" (1908: 58).

In the final analysis, argues Wilson, while 'biologic living' may save a remnant of the White race, for blacks, apparently, there was little hope" (2014: 146). Kellogg was convinced of the possibility that future societies will have so mastered the forces of nature, that disease and degeneracy will have been completely eliminated. Indeed, hospitals and prisons will no longer be required, and the golden age will have finally been restored as the crowning result of human achievement, including obedience to biological laws (Paulson, 1916).

Kellogg's concerns over race degeneration and his ongoing fascination with scientific progress led him into the 'science of eugenics' which he would devote the last 30 years of his life. Eugenics is defined as the "attempt to improve humanity by understanding and systematically controlling hereditary. In 1922 Albert E. Wiggam, journalist, popular speaker, major publicists for eugenic reform, and a close friend of Kellogg, published a book entitled *The New Decalogue of Science*, which became a national best seller. Wiggam's book "called for the replacement of traditional Christianity with the new religion of biology, with eugenics as its centrepiece" (Wilson, 2014: 164). Addressing a fictitious "Statesman," Wiggam stated that in past times God had revealed himself through the Ten Commandments, the Golden Rule, and the Sermon on the Mount, all of which mankind failed to live up to. More recently, however, God had revealed that which was now necessary for modern man to fulfil his obligations to the earlier ethical injunctions: science. Now, "instead of using tablets of stone, burning bushes, prophecies and dreams to reveal His will, He has given men the microscope, the spectroscope, the telescope, the chemist's tube and the statistician's curve in order for men to make their own revelations." In fact, if God's will "is ever to be done on earth as it is in heaven, it will be done through the instrumentalities of science."

Furthermore, if either Christ or Moses were alive today, he "would be the first to perceive that a new Ten Commandments must be added to those on the tables of stone; that a new moral and spiritual dispensation must emerge from the modern Mount Sinai—the laboratory of science." Thus, Wiggam could conclude that "science came not to destroy the great ethical essence of the Bible but to fulfil it. It is the only thing that can fulfil it. And eugenics, which is simply conscious, intelligent organic evolution, furnishes the final program for the completed Christianization of mankind" (cited in Wilson, 2014: 165).

Kellogg could not have agreed more with Wiggam, for he had been searching for decades to discover a "theology of divine immanence that thoroughly divinized biology while at the same time not completely abandoning the ethics of the old faith." It wasn't necessarily a religion to replace Christianity that Kellogg was seeking, rather, "an amplification of the present conception of Christian principles as will make the demands of physical righteousness a part of the greater Decalogue."

From 1916 onwards, Kellogg deemed his mission in the world was to promote "new ethical standards, a new conscience, a broader religion, a code of ethics that will place the canons of biological law alongside those of the Decalogue. Furthermore, it will make man's responsibility to the human race—those who are to come after him, as well as those with whom he comes in contact—the ruling influence of his conduct." Dr J. H. Kellogg believed that along with biologic living, his advancement of eugenics was one of his most important legacies to the betterment of mankind. Just days before he died in 1943, Kellogg wrote that eugenics offers the only hope there is for humanity" (cited in Wilson, 2014: 166–169).

If *Biological Living* represented the core foundation for Dr J. H. Kellogg's health reform ideals, the *Great Controversy Theme* (GCT) constituted the unifying framework for Ellen G. White's philosophy of health, and every other facet of life. It is to this theme (GCT) that the following chapter engages.

4

Ellen G. White's Perspective
on Health Reform

JOHN COBB IN LIVING *Options in Protestant Theology* recognized that all
prominent theologies are constructed on an organizing principle (1962,
12, 121). Such was the centrality of the GCT to her understanding of
the story of salvation that White referred to it over 1,000 times in her
writings. While the GCT did not originate with White, her synthesis of
revealed insights, personal observations, and reading all contributed to
the development of a distinct, coherent, and interconnected Adventist
way of life, which continues today.

For White, the GCT provided the *conceptual key* to understanding
humanity's greatest existential questions: How did life begin? Why does suffering and death occur? Why does good and evil exist? According to White,
the purpose of the Great Controversy is twofold: First, to demonstrate to all
the universe the nature of rebellion initiated originally by Satan in heaven
and in so doing vindicate God's character, and second, to restore the image
of God in fallen humanity (Douglass, 1998: 256). An insight into her understanding of the GCT is portrayed in her book *Patriarchs and Prophets* (338)
where she declares that from the beginning of the "great controversy it has
been Satan's purpose to misrepresent God's character, and to excite rebellion against His law; and this work appears to be crowned with success."
White continues suggesting that myriads of people are seduced by Satan's

deceptions and reject God; however, God's purposes will not be thwarted, for "amid the working of evil, God's purposes move steadily forward to their accomplishment; to all created intelligences He is making manifest His justice and benevolence." Ultimately, in "every age, from midst of apostasy and rebellion, God gathers out a people that are true to Him."

Whilst the saved will ultimately inhabit the New Earth following the millennium in heaven, and will be completely restored in the image of Christ at glorification, or the Second Advent of Christ, the process of restoration commences for the believer in this life. In her book *Education*, White elaborates on, what is for her, *the* core theme of Scripture, stating that the "central theme of the Bible, the theme about which every other in the whole book clusters, is the redemption plan, the *restoration* in the human soul of the image of God . . . . He who grasps this thought has before him an infinite field of study. He has the key that will unlock to him the whole treasurehouse of God's word" (125, 126, emphasis supplied).

Thus, the gospel involves more than the forgiveness of sin; its primary goal is the restoration of God's image in humanity, hence, White unequivocally declares, the "very essence of the gospel is restoration" (DA: 824). Douglass argues, that the vindication of God's justice, fairness and trustworthiness, coupled with the restoration ideal as being central to the gospel ushered in a biblical freshness to White's developing theological system and provided coherence and consistency to all other aspects of her teaching, and this was no more evident than in her approach to health reform (1998: 257).

White's understanding of restoration within the context of the GCT provided the 'mental grid' or 'lens' through which she was able to recognize in the area of disease, and health reform "the fundamental and enduring wisdom of her age, and to reject that which would soon prove worthless" (Douglass, 1998: 278). White's developing notions of health and wholeness were constantly developing. Because of her understanding of the GCT, White saw the implications involved in humanity's indivisible unity of the body, mind, and spirit. Human beings were more than 'free moral agents,' for the interacting, integrating components of mind, body, and spirit required the health of each constituent so that all the components would function effectively. Without the well-being of this synergy, humans would soon suffer and hasten their slide to death (Douglass, 1998: 278).

In a volume of *Testimonies to the Church*, White declares that the "moral powers are weakened, because men and women will not live in obedience to the laws of health and make this great subject a personal duty (3T: 140). While the implications of the GCT concerning health reform and wholeness became increasingly evident in the Adventist movement over time, the journey was not devoid of major tensions along the way for little, if anything, separated the majority of early Adventists from the rest of their American contemporaries concerning a regard for healthful living and wellbeing, including Ellen and James White.

Over a period of 23 years (1848 to 1871), White received five health related visions or dreams. As early as 1848, she was shown the harmful effects of tobacco, coffee, and tea with tobacco, in particular, requiring immediate eradication as the following, unequivocal comment indicates: "I have seen in vision that tobacco was a filthy weed, and that it must be laid aside or given up" (EW: 1Bio: 224). White's clarion calls for ongoing health reform stemmed from pragmatic considerations. Her developing understanding of the mystical, wholistic union between mind and body became extremely practical: "It cannot be to the glory of God for His children to have sickly bodies or dwarfed minds," she declared (3T: 485, 486). In a similar tone, she wrote in *Christ's Object Lessons* that anything, which diminishes physical strength, also enfeebles the mind, making it very difficult to discriminate between right and wrong. "We become less capable of choosing the good, and have less strength of will to do that which we know to be right" (346). Evolving from this theological understanding of wholeness flowed a coherent philosophy of health that was intended to undergird the operation of all SDA health institutions.

Other dietary practices and lifestyle changes were also firmly on the Adventist agenda during the 1850s and 60s including the issue of consumption of swine's flesh. The instruction provided by White was not palatable for many and cut across the regular dietary habits of the majority. In 1854, when modern conveniences were still decades in the future, she called for church members to adopt an attitude and display of cleanliness: "I saw that the houses of the saints should be kept tidy and neat, free from dirt and filth and all uncleanliness." Furthermore, concerning dietary habits, she insisted that believers must take special care of the health that God has provided them, including the discipline to deny an unhealthy appetite, which involved consuming less fine foods, and eating coarse food free from grease. "Then as you sit at the table to eat," she declared, "you can from the heart ask God's blessing upon the food and can derive strength from coarse, wholesome food" (3SM: 274).

The 1863 Otsego Health Vision Essentials

The instruction concerning the health reform principles received by White in 1863 were detailed. Considerable lessons were directed not only towards Adventism in general, but also her husband James and herself, in particular, regarding their ongoing physical welfare (Robinson, 1965: 77). Douglass in *Messenger of the Lord* (1998: 283–284) provides a helpful summary in point form of the core principles contained in White's comprehensive health vision:

- Those who do not control their appetite in eating are guilty of intemperance.
- Swine's flesh is not to be eaten under any circumstance.
- Tobacco in any form is a slow poison.
- Strict cleanliness of the body and home is important.
- Tea and coffee, similar to tobacco, are slow poisons.
- Rich cake, pies, and puddings are injurious.
- Eating between meals injures the stomach and digestive process.
- Adequate time must be allowed between meals, giving the stomach time to rest.
- If a third meal is taken, it should be light and several hours before bedtime.
- People used to meat, gravies, and pastries do not immediately relish a plain, wholesome diet.
- Gluttonous appetite contributes to indulgence of corrupt passions.
- Turning to a plain, nutritious diet may overcome the physical damage caused by the wrong diet.
- Reforms in eating will save expense and labor.
- Children eating flesh meat and spicy foods have strong tendencies toward sexual indulgences.
- Poisonous drugs used as medical prescriptions kill more people than all other causes of death combined.
- Pure water should be used freely in maintaining health and curing illnesses.

- Nature alone has curative powers.
- Common medicines, such as strychnine, opium, calomel, mercury, and quinine, are poisons.
- Parents transmit their weaknesses to their children; prenatal influences are enormous.
- Obeying the laws of health will prevent many illnesses.
- God is often blamed for deaths caused by violation of nature's laws.
- Light and pure air are required, especially in the sleeping quarters.
- Bathing, even a sponge bath, will be beneficial on rising in the morning.
- God will not work healing miracles for those who continually violate the laws of health.
- Many invalids have no physical cause for their illnesses; they have a diseased imagination.
- Cheerful, physical labor will help to create a healthy, cheerful disposition.
- Willpower has much to do with resisting disease and soothing nerves.
- Outdoor exercise is very important to health of mind and body.
- Overwork breaks down both mind and body; routine rest is necessary.
- Many die of diseases caused wholly by eating flesh food.
- All God's promises are given on condition of obedience.
- A healthy mind and body directly affects one's morals and one's ability to discern truth.
- Caring for health is a spiritual matter, reflecting a person's commitment to God.

Arguably one of White's most often cited quotes relates to the essential remedial ingredients of a wholesome lifestyle: "Pure air, sunlight, abstemiousness, rest, exercise, proper diet, the use of water, trust in divine power—these are the true remedies" (MH: 127; 5T: 443). For many Adventists living in 1864, these reform principles were simply too intense. Many of the health principles were certainly not unique to White or Adventists, for other contemporary reformers were promoting similar messages. Indeed, the breadth and depth of the health reform visions astonished White herself, so much so that she wrote: "Many things came directly across my own ideas" (Manuscript 7, 1967).

Bull & Lockhart contend that the Otsego vision in 1863 marked the turning point at which many Seventh-day Adventists began to accept the principles of health. The same authors are also quick to suggest that this did not translate into all Seventh-day Adventists becoming diligent health reformers. "On the contrary, White had to struggle to convince many of her fellow believers to give up their former ways." Interestingly, John Harvey Kellogg was one of a very few, unlike the majority of SDA ministers during this period, who "apparently never wavered in his commitment to health reform . . ." (2007: 165).

While White clearly perceived that the laws of health she received were of divine origin, she was also keenly aware that those same laws were built upon a naturalistic imperative which she called the 'laws of health' that had either been ignored or broken resulting in disease, and as such, the laws of 'cause and effect' were operative. Humanity has violated the laws of health, she noted, and in doing so have run to excess in almost everything. Disease is on the increase, and cause is followed by effect. Many exist in violation to known health laws, and are ignorant of the relationship that their habits of working, eating, and drinking, are exerting on their overall health. "Multitudes remain in inexcusable ignorance in regards to the laws of their being. . . . I have been shown that a great amount of suffering might be saved if all would labor to prevent disease, by strictly obeying the laws of health (4SG: 120, 134, 137, 140). In the same book, White declared that human degeneration results directly from the violation of God's law and the naturalistic laws of health arguing that many marvel that the human race have so degenerated, mentally, morally, and physically, for they "do not understand that it is a violation of God's constitution and laws, and the violation of the laws of health, that has produced this sad degeneracy" (4SG: 124).

Both James and Ellen White acknowledged that Adventist believers would require all the support available in educating themselves concerning the benefits of adopting a healthier lifestyle and the implications for their spiritual wellbeing. James utilized the printed page to draw attention to health matters. In 1864, he would write, "Our people are generally waking up to the subject of health. . . . And they should have publications on the subject to meet their present wants, at prices within the reach of the poorest" (RH, Dec. 13, 1864). Douglass suggests that James White was referring to publications from other contemporary health reformers at the time including, Mann, Trall, Coles, Jackson, Shew, Lewis, Graham, Alcott and others who had been, for years, trying to attract the attention of the general population (1998: 284). While each of the reformers emphasized a particular aspect of health reform, their books were often technical, costly, voluminous, and, at times, "merely personal opinion floating in oceans of verbiage." Furthermore, it appears that none of the reformers had placed healthful living within the context of preparation for the imminent Advent of Christ (Douglass, 1998: 285).

Health Reform and Gospel Commission: An Integrated Perspective

Robinson, in *The Story of Our Health Message*, declares that the outstanding feature of White's 1863 health vision was the merging of spiritual health and physical welfare (1965: 77). Furthermore, this amalgamation of the physical and the spiritual was contextualized within the everlasting gospel commission as depicted in Revelation 14. In *Counsels on Diet and Foods* (32, 33) White indicates the primary purpose in linking the physical and the spiritual on a pragmatic, and experiential level declaring that health reform was a mandatory feature of the third angel's message, and is "just as closely connected with it as are the arm and hand with the human body." She states that it was time for Adventists to act and advance this great work, and that both ministers and people must work in tandem. God's people have a distinct work to do for themselves, and God will not do it for them, and furthermore, "it is an individual work; one cannot do it for another." White sought to persuade the Adventist believers to cleanse themselves from "all filthiness of the flesh and spirit, perfecting holiness in the fear of God," declaring that "gluttony is the prevailing sin of this age," and "lustful appetite makes slaves of men and women, and beclouds their intellects and stupefies their moral sensibilities to such a degree that the sacred, elevated truths of God's word are not appreciated" (CDF: 32, 33).

It is of importance, therefore, to recognize that the major significance for Adventists in White's 1863 vision was not in the general health principles promulgated, for as previously noted, many of these concepts had been well established by other health reformers, rather, it was the recognition that health reforms were part of one's *religious duty* to care for the body in preparation for the soon return of the Lord. The eschatological emphasis is pivotal.

Ginger Hanks-Harwood, in her chapter titled 'Wholeness' in *Remnant and Republic: Adventist Themes for Personal and Social Ethics*, provides an insightful overview of the impact that White's health reform visions, in particular, exerted on future Adventist ideology when stating that 1863 marked the year when Seventh-day Adventists began to promulgate a wholistic view of the individual. The view that the body, mind, and spirit are all integrated and interrelated constituent elements that together form a single being is the very cornerstone on which Adventism rests. Believing that these three are interdependent and constantly interacting, SDAs have adopted a 'systems' approach in their anthropology, meaning that "the whole person cannot be understood merely as a sum of separate, constituent parts (1995: 127, 128).

White's counsel was intended to be both specific and practical as she sought to apply the principles of the GCT in a wholistic context—the spiritual, the mental and the physical. Locating health matters within the context of eschatological expectations (Revelation 14) raised health issues from matters of mere personal opinion to the level of spiritual commitment and character development (Douglass, 1998: 292). While the linking of health reform and the restoration of humanity with the gospel appeared a strange mix for many, White was convinced that an individual's state of health affected their spiritual commitment, growth and discernment. Unambiguously, she deemed that the adoption of true health reform principles was integral to a sanctified life, and preparation for heavenly translation. In 1867, she wrote that Adventists have a work to do for themselves, which they should not leave for God to do for them.

For White *restoration*, the goal of the GCT, is again, very apparent concerning the state of God's people when Christ returns, for when He returns to earth, He comes "not to cleanse us from our sins, to remove from us the defects in our characters, or to cure us of the infirmities of our tempers and dispositions." She continues, declaring that "if wrought for us at all, this work will be accomplished *before that time*" for when the Lord returns, those who are holy will remain holy, and those who have "preserved their bodies and spirits in holiness, in sanctification and honor, will then receive the finishing touches of immortality (2T: 355, emphasis supplied).

J. H. Waggoner, an SDA leader, and contemporary with James and Ellen White, speaking on behalf of the fledgling Adventist movement, articulated well the overall impact of White's health reform emphasis, particularly the theme of restoration. He declared that Adventists do not profess to be pioneers in the general principles of the health reform for the "facts on which this movement is based have been elaborated, in a great measure, by reformers, physicians, and writers on physiology and hygiene, and so may be found scattered through the land." As mere hygienic and physiological truths, they might be examined by some at their leisure, and yet others will deem them of minor consequence; however, "when placed on a level with the great truths of the third angel's message by the sanction and authority of God's Spirit, and so declared to be the means whereby a weak people may be made strong to overcome, and our diseased bodies cleansed and fitted for translation, then it comes to us as an essential part of present truth, to be received with the blessing of God, or rejected at our peril (RH, 1866: 7, cited in Robinson, 1965: 79, 80).

Health Science

Authors, Stoy and Leilani Proctor in *Searching for the Fountain of Youth* perceptively articulated the results from the advancement of health reform within Adventism arguing that the health and lifespan advantages of Adventists have been traced to the way they live and eat. Since the mid-nineteenth century they have practiced eight secrets of health that reduce their risk of cancer, and heart disease which are the two leading causes of premature death. By limiting the impact of these two potentially fatal killers, Seventh-day Adventists enjoy superior health and longevity than the general population. Their health foundations have now been supported, in general, by scientific confirmation, so how did they know before the scientists? The authors concur that it emanated from a woman named Ellen G. White, who believed that God did not want people to suffer unnecessary illness and death, but instead, enjoy maximum wellness. White wrote with "amazing simplicity and accuracy what has since been proved to be the best formula for health and longevity" (1991).

Also of interest are a series of long-term medical research projects conducted by Loma Linda University in Riverside, California during the past 40 years. Two studies on Adventist health involving 24,000 and 34,000 Californian Adventists were conducted seeking to measure the link between Seventh-day Adventist lifestyle, diet, disease and mortality. Due in part to their unique dietary habits, Adventists exhibit a consistently lower risk than other Americans of suffering from certain diseases. These ongoing studies provide a unique opportunity to answer scientific questions about how diet and other health habits affect the risk of suffering from many chronic diseases. Although not sponsored by the denomination's administrative body, the church is supportive of the studies, which have of more recent times become the subject of significant national media coverage in America through established media outlets such as ABC News, *World News Tonight*, and *Good Morning America*.

In the November 2005 edition of the *National Geographic magazine*, the feature article titled "Longevity: The Secrets of a Long Life" included recognition that SDAs in the Loma Linda, California, region "rank among America's longevity all-stars." Researchers discovered that residents from Sardinia, Italy, the islands of Okinawa, Japan and Loma Linda, California "produce a high rate of centenarians, suffer a fraction of the diseases that commonly kill people in other parts of the developed world, and enjoy more healthy years of life. In sum, they offer three sets of "best practices" to emulate. The first major study of Adventists commenced in 1960, and became known as the *Adventist Mortality Study*. This research involved 22,940 California Adventists, and entailed an intensive 5-year follow-up and a more informal 25-year follow-up. The results were significant indeed:

- Death rates from all cancers was 60% lower for Adventist men and 76% lower for Adventist women

- Lung cancer 21% lower

- Colorectal cancer 62% lower

- Breast cancer 85% lower

- Coronary heart disease 66% lower for Adventist men, 98% lower for Adventist women.

Two more major health and lifestyle studies have taken place since the initial research in 1960. Adventist Health Study 1 (AHS-1) was conducted between 1974 and 1988 and the data from the study is numerous, linking diet to cancer and coronary heart disease. AHS-2 commenced in 2002 and continues into the present, exploring the links between lifestyle, diet and disease among the broader base of Seventh-day Adventists in America and Canada. This study, which is funded by the National Cancer Institute in America, was awarded a $5.5 million grant in July 2011, by the National Institutes of Health to continue the study (http://www.llu.edu/public-health/health/future.page).

One might assume that the scientific research impulse within Adventism is a recent phenomenon. In spite of the fact that people in America during much of the nineteenth century saw no connection between disease and lifestyle, both White and Kellogg became convinced of the link. We have already observed White's understanding, and recognition that health reforms formed an integral part of the believer's *religious duty* to care for the body in preparation for the impending Parousia. What is less obvious, however, is the major contribution that Dr. J. H. Kellogg afforded Adventism by providing the initial scientific basis supporting White's health reform agenda. Before Kellogg's contribution to Adventist Health Reform is assessed, a brief digression into the nature of prejudice and fanaticism associated with prophetic voices, and visions is warranted.

Visions, Fanaticism, and Prejudice

If the source of White's visions continue to defy consensus today, it was no different to the views of her own generation. While the majority of contemporary Adventists continue to maintain that her revelations were authentic and divinely inspired, numerous detractors would argue otherwise, offering a variety of explanations other than a divine source, including hysteria, mesmerism, hypnotism, catalepsy and hallucinations among others (Ferret, 2008: 56, 57). Prophetic manifestations within the Millerite movement tended to exist primarily on the periphery and were often associated with fanaticism (Burt, 2002: 12). William Miller and his associates were very conscious of the "movement's fanatical potential" (Knight, 1993: 172). In his 1843, New Year's address, Miller issued a direct warning to his followers declaring that Satan's desire is to defeat the true believers by "scattering coals of wild fire among you; for if he cannot drive you into disbelief and doubt, he will try his wild fire of fanaticism" (ST, Jan. 25: 150). Burt contends that while Miller and others preached the Advent message, the movement also attracted the more demonstrative and experiential traditions, particularly the Methodists and the Christian churches (2002: 55). While these demonstrative expressions did not originate with Millerism, they certainly reflected the religious background of its adherents (Ferret, 2006: 57). In her book, *Fits, Trances, and Visions: Experiencing Religion and Explaining Experience from Wesley to James*,

Ann Taves argues that religious demonstrations in revival meetings were widespread and involved both genders, where weeping, bodily contortions, shouting, and fainting were commonplace, accompanied at times by dreams and visions (1999: 153–161).

While revelations, visions and demonstrative experiences were in vogue for many in the religious sphere, these phenomena certainly did not receive unanimous support throughout the Christian world at the time, let alone their secular counterparts. Miller's reasoning that the anticipated Second Advent would transpire around 1843 was not based on charismatic revelations, but instead, via reasoned logic supported by the motto, 'prove all things and hold fast to that which is good.' Furthermore, Miller's biblical conclusions concerning the nature and timing of the imminent parousia were not conceived by chance, as he was determined to follow the Barconian injunction to "proceed regularly and gradually from one axiom to another," for it was Barconianism, in a religious context, which became identified with the *sola scriptura* principle or the Bible alone, a Reformation legacy. Miller was determined to lay aside all prepossessions, and thoroughly compare Scripture with Scripture, and to pursue its study in a methodical manner (Bull & Lockhart, 2007: 26, 27). Ferret suggests that Miller's philosophy was reasonably simple: reason always came first for it alone expounded the Bible and visions were secondary (2006: 58).

The months, indeed years following the disappointment of 1844 witnessed intense psychological and spiritual trauma for many former Millerites. To the public and the scoffing religious world, they became targets for innuendos and negative insinuations (Scharnborst, 1994: 28–41). Charismatic phenomena including both visions and revelations were considered suspect and highly controversial, particularly by the former Millerites (Arthur L. White, 1969: 31). The now defunct Millerite movement along with the emergent Seventh-day Adventists continued to be considered suspect, both by rival churches, and the general populace, who became increasingly prejudiced against religious groups who featured a charismatic figure within their midst proclaiming guidance through divinely inspired visionary experiences.

'Fanatics' became a derogatory term employed to summarize such movements, and it would appear that the difficult lot of the biblical prophet, and mid-nineteenth-century America appeared somewhat similar (Ferret, 2008: 60). In hindsight, the year 1844 was indeed an eventful one, not only for the disappointed Millerites, but also other prophetic figures including the Mormon prophet, Joseph Smith, who was killed by a mob in the city of Illinois (Knight, 1999: 36).

While the title 'religious fanatics' was quick and easy to impose; the stigma associated with the label would take much longer to eradicate. In relation to health and medical practice, as noted previously, 'quackery' became the catchphrase of the day. Health educator Dr. M. G. Hardinge summarizes the age appropriately when suggesting that it was "a time of great confusion and medical ignorance in which orthodox medicine and quackery worked side by side, each mixing a little bit of truth with plenty of unadulterated nonsense" (Coon, 1993: 12).

Ellen White was acutely aware of the toxic impact that extremist views exerted on the Adventist movement, particularly in elevating prejudice. She argued that it was time that something was done to avert novices from advocating health reform for they do more injury than the most intelligent, and wise men, with the best influence they can exert, can counteract. "It is impossible," she declared, for the greatest qualified health reform advocates to "fully relieve the minds of the public from the prejudice received through the wrong course of these extremists," and to situate the important subject of health reform upon a correct basis in the communities where these men have figured. The most valuable truths are cast aside by the people as unworthy of a hearing. White concludes stating that these people are referred to as "representatives of health reformers and Sabbath-keepers in general. A great responsibility rests upon those who have thus proved a stumbling-block to unbelievers" (2T: 386, 387).

In the *Review and Herald* edition of March 17, 1868, James White recognized well the problems associated with extremist views and the ongoing challenges this brought to his wife's counsel and role. "She works to this disadvantage namely: she makes strong appeals to the people, which a few feel deeply, and take strong positions, and go to extremes. Then so save the cause from ruin in consequence of these extremes, she is obliged to come out with reproofs for extremists in a public manner." James then exposes the dilemma stating that what Ellen "may say to urge the tardy, is taken by the prompt to urge them over the mark. And what she may say to caution the prompt, zealous, incautious ones is taken by the tardy as an excuse to remain too far behind."

Thus, fanaticism and extremism was as rife in the nineteenth-century American health reform movement as in any other movement, and when Adventism's focus was directed towards health reform including the establishing of SDA health institutions in the 1870s on the basis on Ellen White's visions, the same stigma was evident in society as was previously witnessed following the Millerite disappointment.

The Battle Creek Sanitarium:
An Experiment with a Scientific Basis

The Battle Creek Sanitarium which commenced in 1866 was originally known as the Western Health Reform Institute in response to recommendations from White who was convinced that it was now appropriate for Adventists to establish their own health institution based on the true pattern of healthful living revealed to her in vision, and that the care of the infirmed must be in harmony with those newly revealed principles (Schwarz, 2006: 62).

The impetus for this institutional development was in no small part a result of a reflective process following treatment received by James White at 'Our Home,' a health institution at Dansville, New York, directed by Dr. Jackson. 'Our Home' was recognized for its hydropathic treatments and application of natural treatments and remedies rather than conventional drug therapy, so widespread at the time. James White was an extremely active man in the Adventist cause. He was a pioneer of the Seventh-day Adventist movement, instrumental in its organisation, and carried the burden of financial accountability in the face of continual reluctance from others. His incessant pen provided clarity, doctrinal unity, and encouragement for the emerging movement. While Ellen received the heavenly guidance concerning the future Adventist sojourn on earth, James was instrumental in bringing those revelations to fruition through his immense organizational skills. In spite of his enormous contribution to his church, James did not know how to rest, nor was he self-controlled in his dietary habits. He carried the workload of several men, and by age 44 his body was simply 'worn out.' On one occasion, Ellen penned the following words to her husband in a personal letter:

> All the powers on earth could not help you unless you work in harmony, exercising your reason and your judgment and setting aside your feelings and your inclination. You are in a critical condition. (3 Bio: 82)

Mental and physical exhaustion is believed to have contributed to James's first stroke on August 16, 1865, resulting in almost complete incapacitation. His inability to respond to rest whilst at home led Ellen to consider other remedial options; eventually resulting in a decision to visit Dr. Jackson's hydrotherapy institution in Dansville approximately a month following James's declining condition. Ellen White was convinced that 'water-cure' therapies were part of the recently revealed health reform principles. Interestingly, the Whites were required to defend their attendance at the Dansville retreat from some zealous church members who insisted that trust in God and prayer were alone, adequate. In a muted rebuke, Ellen White responded declaring that while we did not feel like despising the means the Lord had positioned in our reach for the recovery of health, we believed that God was above all, and it was He who had provided water as His agent would have to use it to assist abused nature to recover her exhausted energies. "We believed God would bless the efforts we were making in the direction of health" (RH, Feb. 20, 1866).

Recognizing no appreciable improvement in James's condition following three months of treatment at Dansville, Ellen opted to return home to Battle Creek. While she insisted that the Dansville experience was not in vain, and that there was much to commend concerning health reform, she was also quick to declare that "some of the principles that were advocated there were contrary to the teachings of Christ," and furthermore, some of the medical advice afforded her husband "might well have proved fatal . . ." (Robinson, 1965: 135). She summed up their sojourn at Dansville with a mixed response stating that while they "did not receive all the ideas and sentiments and suggestions advanced," we did "gather many things of value from those who had obtained an experience in health reform. We did not feel that there was any necessity of gathering the chaff with the wheat" (1MS: 1867).

Examples of the 'chaff' that White referred to included Dr. Jackson's insistence that salt should be discarded totally; a lack of fresh air in the facilities which impacted James ability to recover; the Whites were deemed to be too religious and this contributed to James's invalid condition; the insistence by the Dansville physicians that James be totally immobilized (physical and mental inaction) was viewed by Ellen as the greatest obstacle to her husband's recovery. Of immense negative significance was the fact that the Dansville treatment regime emphasized amusements and pleasure, card playing and dancing, theatre attendance etc., which, as far as the Whites' were concerned, could not be harmonized with the teachings of the New Testament Scriptures (RH, Feb 20. 1866). Thus, while stating that the Dansville hydrotherapy establishment was one of the best of its kind in America, Ellen was adamant that Seventh-day Adventists must not be naïve regarding the nature of contemporary health reform institutions and their treatment regimes.

Maintaining Adventism's sectarian perspective, White reminded her church that it had been revealed to her that those who are stoutly fortified with religious principles and are unyielding in obedience to all God's requirements cannot receive benefits from the popular health institutions of the day that others of a different faith can, for "Sabbathkeepers are singular in their faith." To uphold all of God's commandments as He requires in order to be owned and approved of Him is extremely difficult in popular water cures. "They have to carry along with them at all times the gospel sieve and sift everything they hear, that they may choose the good and refuse the bad" (1T: 489). The implications of this comment continue to be experienced within contemporary Adventism.

A further vision received in Rochester on December 25, 1865 both confirmed and re-emphasized the significance of the relationship between health reform and the gospel in the context of the third angel's message. Robinson notes that the Rochester vision was supplementary to, yet perhaps equal with the 1863, Otsego vision. While the first revelation established the health principles and urged their adoption by the church, the second pointed out that the response to the initial health reform principles had been disappointing and had fallen short of what is should have been, and it also made more clear the relation of that reform to the gospel message to be given to the world (1965: 140).

The same vision also revealed that SDAs must develop their own health institutions, as this would provide a means of introducing the Adventist faith in new contexts and raising the "standard of truth where it would have been impossible to gain access had not prejudice been removed" (1T: 493). Furthermore, the "great object" of Adventist institutions "is not only health, but perfection and the spirit of holiness, which cannot be attained with diseased bodies and minds" (1T: 554).

When the Western Health Reform Institute opened its doors in 1866 under the supervision of Dr. H. S. Lay, one patient was registered, while the staff consisted of two doctors, two bath attendants, one untrained nurse, three or four helpers, several inconveniences and a large measure of faith

(Schwarz, 2006: 62; Robinson, 1965: 153). Four months later, every room in the three buildings was occupied; however, financial challenges were always present with debt a common companion. Largely through the influence of the White's, the Institute modified its financial base resulting in its reclassification as a 'non-profit organisation.' By 1873, the Institute's financial operations had improved significantly along with its growing reputation. The influence of *The Health Reformer*, under the editorship of James White had successfully rebounded from a period of instability, caused primarily because of extremist views promoted by the former editor, Dr. R. S. Trall. James White, in his first editorial was quick to declare the purpose of the paper insisting that its purpose was to reach the communities "with all their prejudices, and their ignorance of the laws of life, where they are." James continued arguing that the *Reformer* "will avoid extreme positions, and come as near those who need reforming as possible, and yet be true to the principles of health reform" (*Health Reformer*, March, 1871).

As a result of James White's editorial experience and leadership, membership subscriptions in the first year rose from 3,000 to over 10,000. Furthermore, the widening influence of the paper was drawing many patients who had both the means to pay for treatment and also possessed considerable influence in their respective communities (Robinson, 1965: 202, 203). It also became increasingly evident; however, that a groundswell of negative opinion concerning the medical integrity of the Institute was emerging. Robinson cites one such response, as an example: "Your publishing buildings and your college are first class, but your health department is third rate." Patients would remain at the facility for a few days and then leave, disappointed with the facilities, building and physicians. To clarify, there was never a shortage of patients, however, a high proportion of those who occupied the rooms did not have the resources to fund their stay and were, therefore, accepted at reduced rates, placing further stress on the Institutes already feeble resources. This was of major concern to the White's and in May 1877, James White shared their concerns declaring that they were now satisfied that our health institute could "not rise to eminence and the full measure of usefulness without thoroughly educated physicians to stand at the head of it. We laid plans to gain this point" (RH, May, 24, 1877).

Robinson, when taking into account Adventism's sectarian positioning in society at the time, including prejudicial attitudes towards both the movement and visionary experiences in general, declares that scientific advances required a different strategy. "The cause of health reform might well be begun by discarding the use of drugs, adopting a rational diet, and using water and other natural agencies as remedies for disease," he argues, but it was unfeasible to make a solid appeal in its behalf to the more cultured and educated classes of society until "there was a leadership whose *scientific knowledge could command respect*. The benefits of rational treatment had been demonstrated empirically, but this was not sufficient. *The scientific and physiological principles for the success of certain rational and therapeutic agencies must be made clear*" (Robinson, 1965: 204; emphasis mine).

Clearly, the physicians and medical staff at the Health Reform Institute were lacking in basic scientific knowledge that was considered, not only necessary for the proper diagnosis and treatment of the many presenting diseases, but also mandatory in view of the burgeoning scientific date now available to both physicians and the common person. Again, Robinson's (1965: 204) evaluation of the precarious situation confronting the Institute appears accurate when observing that it was impossible for the Health Reform Institute to acquire favorable recognition among the finest and most progressive members of the medical profession while some of the physicians on the staff were originally equipped for their service with a few months of training at the most. If they were to persist with a critical attitude concerning the practice of the physicians, they must be able to bring to the discussion of their points of difference "*a storehouse of scientific knowledge* of chemistry, anatomy, and physiology. They must be able to *keep abreast of the important medical discoveries* that were being made at this time" (emphasis mine.)

Undoubtedly, a major dilemma facing the Seventh-day Adventist church in the mid-1800s and beyond was overcoming prejudice. How do the Sabbath keeping Adventists, who have worn the rebuke, scoffing and prejudiced attitudes of society for several decades following the Millerite disappointment, now engage in a meaningful way with their communities? Behavioral change can be effected immediately; attitudinal change can take generations. One thing is certain; people cannot relate to or accommodate too much change all at once.

The early Adventists proclaimed and sought to keep holy the seventh-day Sabbath when a regular six-day working week was in vogue, and where Sabbath day exemptions were nigh impossible (Douglass, 1998: 282). Furthermore, many people personally remembered, or at least had heard 'second hand' about the clarion call of the Millerite adherents, to exit 'Babylon' and join the only true believers in readiness for the literal appearance of Christ to earth; all of which appeared both suspect, and far-fetched, particularly when the predicted event did not materialize. The average American at the time was not interested in hearing about the supposed rationale for the non-return of Christ, or the personal stories of the disappointed in their midst; instead, they simply consigned these individuals and the movement to the 'fanaticism bin.'

Ellen White, more than anyone, understood the immense challenges facing her church concerning ongoing prejudice in connection with the development of their own health institution. She declared that the health institution would hopefully provide "the means of introducing our faith in new places and raising the standard of truth where it would have been impossible to gain access had not prejudice first been removed" (1T: 485–495, 553–564, 612–620).

One of the major reasons as to why White's health reform visions were not deemed sufficient or adequate on their own to propel the re-form agenda to the point of wide acceptance within society was based on perceived fanaticism and continuing prejudiced attitudes towards vi-sions. While White's integration of health reform with the mission of the Adventist church made it possible for Adventists to seize the initiative in combining health with faith in the context of religious duty, it was Dr. J. H. Kellogg's commitment to the progressive nature of scientific and medi-cal advances that provided a solid theoretical basis undergirding White's health reform visions (Reid, 1993: 91).

At the annual meeting of the Health Reform Institute in 1876, Kel-logg, just 24 years old, became medical superintendent. James White was elated with the decision, and the following words express his hopes for a positive future. "We have never seen as bright a prospect of success before our health institute as at the present time." Plans had been in place for more than five years to attain the benefits of the highest, most meticu-lously educated and cultivated medical talent in the nation, and God has helped in this work this far, and "we trust His help to its full completion" (RH, October, 19, 1876).

Thus began, Robinson writes, "a new era in the health reform move-ment among Seventh-day Adventists. The leadership of members of the medical profession, more highly trained in scientific lines, resulted not so much in altering the principles upon which the work had been carried forward for a decade as to *justify* these principles" by providing satisfactory motive for their "adoption in the treatment of the sick and the education of all (1965: 211).

Dr. J. H. Kellogg's greatest desire was to turn the poorly equipped Institute "into a scientifically respectable institution where a wide variety of medical and surgical techniques could be used" (Numbers, 2008: 181). He had the full support of Ellen and James White and immediately set out to ally himself with them in their efforts to maintain control of the rapidly growing organisation. Reid states "John Harvey Kellogg was the ideal man to lead the advance for his close association with the Whites gave him authority in the church." Furthermore, his "support of the principles of health reform as taught by the church provided contact for his efforts, and his regular medical training in one of the nation's finest schools gave him a clear connection with advancing scientific medicine" (1982: 150). Indeed, the young Kellogg also had a right to feel somewhat proud, as he was the first SDA to receive the title of M.D. He along with Ellen White resented having those not of the faith, "sneeringly [assert] that those who believe present truth are weak-minded, deficient in education, without position or influence." Furthermore, a "first- rate medical center would prove her detractors wrong and bring fame and honor to Seventh-day Adventists" (Numbers, 2008: 181).

Kellogg studied, researched, spoke and wrote about almost any topic that could be included under the umbrella of healthful living. Michael O'Donnell, an editor of the *American Journal of Health promotion*, defined health promotion as the "science and art of helping people change their lifestyle to move toward a state of optimal health. Optimal health is defined as a balance of physical, emotional, social, spiritual and intellectual health" (Nieman, 1992: 123). Willis argues that in light of O'Donnell's definition, there can be "little doubt that . . . that Dr John Harvey Kellogg made a profound—and probably unsurpassed—contribution to health promotion" (2003: 99). Dr Gertrude Brown was adamant declaring that health promotion was not Kellogg's work; rather, "it was his way of life!" (Willis, 2003: 100). Kellogg's 'biological living' or 'optimal health' was "utopian thinking at its very best" (Willis, 2003: 100). Following his death, the Seventh-day Adventist church, whom he had served for many years, through his scientific underpinning of the health reform agenda published the following obituary in the *Review and Herald*, 1943:

> Throughout his entire medical career Doctor Kellogg was a pioneer in the promotion of the principles of health and temperance.

He did much in the field of medical research and the development of therapeutic principles and methods. Thousands are indebted to him for the benefits they received from his medical journals, books, lectures, and personal service as a physician. His death marks the passing of a great man in the field he occupied.

If Ellen White's health related visions provided the principles for reform, it was Kellogg's initiatives that provided the scientific corroboration and institutional structures to undergird those principles. In the process, however, it became increasingly obvious that Ellen White and Dr. John H. Kellogg's understanding of the nature of institutionalized health reform and how those reforms should be implemented were following different trajectories; a divergence that continues to exist to the present day.

5

Ellen G. White and
the Medical Missionary Model

HEALTH REFORM WAS SUCH a major concern to Ellen White that it occupied more of her literary time and consumed more writers' ink than
any other single theme. For over fifty years, her counsel was addressed to
physicians, ministers, institutional managers and her church in general.
While much of her instruction gave direction to the SDA medical work
in general, other specific counsel was provided at crucial times as the
medical work advanced (MM: x).

Whereas White is normally associated with Seventh-day Adventist
health reform, it is Joseph Bates, as noted previously, who was the first of the
fledgling movement to adopt principles of health reform, prior to the Great
Disappointment of 1844. Nonetheless, it was White who was responsible
for the "direct connection between Adventism and health" (Jackson, 2015:
21). Following the Great Disappointment, Bates was reluctant to share his
focus on health principles lest they detract from preaching the imminent
return of Christ. White, similarly to Bates, did not envisage health reform
as a priority as the Sabbatarian Adventists struggled to make sense of their
fractured world, and it was not until 1848, that White in vision, was first
introduced to basic health principles which were initially limited to the ad-
verse effects of tea, coffee, and tobacco (Robinson, 1965: 65–72).

In 1866, White earnestly urged Adventists to place a higher estimate upon the divine instruction provided concerning health principles. She singled out the ministry, in particular, exhorting them to not only adopt health principles in their totality but also to elaborate on those principles in their churches. "One important part of the work of ministry is to faithfully present to the people the health reform, as it stands connected with the third angel's message, as a part and parcel of the same work. They should not fail to adopt it for themselves, and should urge it upon all who profess to believe the truth" (1T: 466–470). White insisted that the work of reform had "scarcely been entered upon yet," and that few Adventists understood "how much their habits of diet have to do with their health, their characters, *their usefulness in the world*, and their eternal destiny" (1T: 485, 488, 489, emphasis supplied).

Jackson argues that the motivations for health reform are what differentiate White from her contemporaries. "While recognizing God's hand in natural laws like Graham, Alcott, and Coles, White does not suggest that health laws are equal to the Ten Commandments, nor that obedience to health law brings about salvation, or the millennium" (2015: 23). As noted previously, White, in 1863 provided the link between health and spiritual experience declaring that it was a sacred obligation to attend to our health, and awaken others to their duty (3SM: 280). Thus was born the foundation of a health program that today spans the globe. The implications of White's health reform directives have witnessed the development and growth of institutions stressing the importance of medical education to better comprehend and propagate health principles, and in doing do, complete man's sacred duties in relation to health (Jackson, 2015: 24).

It is rarely proposed that any doctrine, teaching or policy be established on a single text, comment or recommendation, nor seldom does an idea, theory or narrative arrive fully developed and functionally cohesive. There is always an introductory phase featuring a range of undefined discussion, and explanations that appear only partial, while documentation is often sparse and incomplete. In other words, as Fielder perceptively observes, "the table must be set before dinner is served" (2012: 45).

There was a time when 'medical missionaries' did not feature in Adventist discussions. Instead, survival, doctrinal formulations, and organizational expansion consumed the bulk of the movement's time, energy and resources during the first three decades of existence. The phrase, 'medical missionaries' first appeared in the *Review and Herald* in November 1883 and was later included in *Testimonies for the Church*, vol. 6, published in 1901. Prior to this, the terms 'Christian help work,' or 'benevolent work' were employed (Fielder, 2012: 46). Overall, White utilized the term 'medical missionary' 2,532 times throughout her published writings. In January 1891, White wrote concerning the broader needs for trained missionaries to gain access to unbelievers and reduce prejudice:

> How shall the Lord's work be done? How can we gain access to souls buried in midnight darkness? Prejudice must be met; corrupt religion is hard to deal with. The very best ways and means of work must be prayerfully considered. There is a way in which many doors will be opened to the missionary. Let him become intelligent in the care of the sick, as a nurse, or how to treat disease, as a physician, and if he is imbued with the spirit of Christ, what a field of uselfulness is opened before him. (CH: 33)

Regarding the need for medical missionaries in the cities, she wrote, "there should be corps of organized, well-disciplined workers; not merely one or two, but scores should be set to work" (MM: 300). White continued her counsel stating that she had been shown that in "our labor for the enlightenment of the people in the large cities the work has not been as well organized or the methods of labor as efficient as in other churches that have not the great light we regard as so essential." She then provides the answer: "Why is this? Because so many of our laborers have been those who love to preach (and many who were not thoroughly qualified to preach were set at work), and a large share of the labor has been put forth in preaching" (MM: 301).

The call for adequate training of medical missionaries was made abundantly clear when White penned a letter from Australia, dated September 16, 1892 stating the she was perplexed regarding several matters concerning the education of men and women to become medical missionaries:

> I am deeply interested in the subject of medical missionary work and the education of men and women for that work. I could wish that there were one hundred nurses in training where there is one. It ought to be thus. Both men and women can be so much more useful as medical missionaries than as missionaries without the medical education. I am more and more impressed with the fact that a more decided testimony must be borne upon this subject, that more direct efforts must be made to interest the proper persons, setting before them the advantages that every missionary will have in understanding how to treat those who are diseased in

body, as well as to minister to sin-sick souls. This double ministra-
tion will give the laborer together with God access to homes, and
will enable him to reach all classes of society. (CH: 503)

White continued suggesting, "both men and women can be more useful as
medical missionaries than as missionaries without a medical education,"
and in the same letter emphasized the value of the medical missionary in
comparison to preaching the gospel alone:

> I have been surprised at being asked by physicians if I did not
> think it would be more pleasing to God for them to give up their
> medical practice and enter the ministry. I am prepared to answer
> such an inquirer: If you are a Christian and a competent physi-
> cian, you are qualified to do tenfold more good as a missionary
> for God than if you were to go forth merely as a preacher of the
> word. (CH: 502–504)

Turning her attention specifically to the responsibilities of physicians in the
book, *Medical Ministry*, she declared:

> Every medical practitioner, whether he acknowledges it or not, is
> responsible for the souls as well as the bodies of his patients. The
> Lord expects of us much more than we often do for Him. Every
> physician should be a devoted, intelligent gospel medical mission-
> ary, familiar with Heaven's remedy for the sin-sick soul as well as
> with the science of healing bodily disease. (MM: 31)

White spoke of the need for a medical-ministry approach in health
care that emphasized a combined ministry to both soul and body. It was
to be wholistic in all aspects. Citing Christ, as the ultimate expression of
God's love towards humanity, she declared, "Christ stands before us as
the pattern Man, the great Medical Missionary—an example for all who
should come after" (MM: 20). What, then, White asks, "is the example
that we are to set to the world?" The answer: "We are to do the same
work that the great Medical Missionary undertook in our behalf. We are
to follow the path of self-sacrifice trodden by Christ (MM: 20). "Christ,
not only preached the word, but also relieved suffering through healing,"
White insists, and for this reason "the Lord has marked out a way in which
His people are to carry forward a work of physical healing combined with
the teaching of the word" (MM: 14).

While the charge for the medical missionary is to follow Christ's example of self-sacrifice, one might also enquire as to whether God expects

His followers to perform miraculous healings as did Christ when on earth as part of doing the same great work of Jesus. White seemingly anticipated this question and responded in the early pages of *Medical Ministry*:

> The way in which Christ worked was to preach the word, and to re-lieve suffering by miraculous works of healing. But I am instructed that we cannot now work in this way; for Satan will exercise his power by working miracles. God's servants today could not work by means of miracles, because spurious works of healing, claiming to be divine, will be wrought. (MM: 14)

White was convinced that in her day, reformation was to precede miracle working:

> You may say, "Why not, then, take hold of the work, and heal the sick as Christ did?" I answer, You are not ready. Some have believed; some have been healed; but there are many who make themselves sick by intemperate eating or by indulging in other wrong habits. When they get sick, shall we pray for them to be raised up, that they may carry on the very same work again? There must be a reformation throughout our ranks; the people must reach a higher standard before we can expect the power of God to be manifested in a marked manner for the healing of the sick . . . (MM: 15)

It would appear that the way forward for Adventists in the nineteenth century was not to pursue miraculous healings, which could be satanically inspired but rather through educative processes:

> Jesus Christ is the Great Healer, but He desires that by living in conformity with His laws we may cooperate with Him in the re-covery and the maintenance of health. Combined with the work of healing there must be an imparting of knowledge of how to resist temptations. Those who come to our sanitariums should be aroused to a sense of their own responsibility to work in harmony with the God of truth. (MM: 13)

White argued that the establishment of sanitariums was a divinely inspired process, which would provide for healing of both body and spirit, and fur-thermore, to integrate medical institutions with medical missionaries:

> For this reason the Lord has marked out a way in which His people are to carry forward a work of physical healing combined with the teaching of the word. Sanitariums are to be established, and with these institutions are to be connected workers who will carry forward genuine medical missionary work. Thus a guarding

influence is thrown around those who come to the sanitariums for treatment. This is the provision the Lord has made whereby gospel medical missionary work is to be done for many souls. These institutions are to be established out of the cities, and in them educational work is to be intelligently carried forward. (MM: 14)

White continued by declaring that the highest aim for any Seventh-day Adventist worker in the church's medical institutions involved both a spiritual and evangelistic work:

The highest aim of the workers in these institutions is to be the spiritual health to the patients. Successful evangelistic work can be done in connection with medical missionary work. It is as these lines of work are united that we may expect to gather the most precious fruit for the Lord. (MM: 26)

With the launching of the journal *Medical Ministry* in 1891, Seventh-day Adventists members were kept informed of the importance of the medical missionary model in health care. Under the title "The Christian Physician as a Missionary," White, as noted above, elaborated on the responsibilities of all church members to engage in home missionary work (Robinson, 1965: 271).

The importance for each minister and church member to be engaged in some capacity in medical missionary work, in the mind of White, cannot be underestimated. During the late 1890s when tensions between Dr. J. H. Kellogg and the Adventist ministry were becoming more noticeable, she made the following observations:

Some have looked upon the medical missionary work with suspicion because of its constantly increasing success. Unless these are baptized with the Holy Spirit they will continue to entertain their jealous feelings, whatever power God may reveal in advancing the truth. They will lose the spiritual blessings they might have had and will bring the divine judgments upon themselves. The truth which is a savor of life unto life, if received, becomes, when rejected, a means of hardening the heart. (Letter 233, 1899; 21MR: 401)

White was determined to point out that the medical missionary work be assigned a higher priority than was currently manifested. "Again and again the Lord has pointed out the work which the church in Battle Creek and those all through America are to do," for the "medical missionary workers are doing the long-neglected work which God gave to the church in Battle Creek. . . ." and the "Lord says to the presidents of conferences and to other influential brethren: "Remove the stumbling blocks that have been placed before the people." She continues her strong indictment stating that the Lord has "moved upon Dr. Kellogg and his associates to do the work which be-longs to the church and which was offered to them, but which they did not choose to accept" (8T: 70–71). "If the medical missionary workers will carry this line of effort into the churches everywhere, if they will work in the fear of God, they will find many doors opened before them, and angels will work with them" (8T: 72). Concluding her comments, White cautions that when the "Lord moves upon the churches, bidding them do a certain work, and they refuse to do that work; and when some, their human efforts united with the divine, endeavor to reach to the very depths of human woe and misery, God's blessing will rest richly upon them (8T: 72).

The issues facing the churches concerning the medical missionary work were quite substantial, so much so, that the italics are not supplied; they are in the original:

> This work is the work the churches have left undone, and *they can-not prosper until they have taken hold of this work in the cities, in highways, and in hedges.* Then angels of God will co-operate with human instrumentalities, and a religious system will be inaugu-rated to relieve the necessities of suffering human beings who are in physical, mental, and moral need. (HM, Nov. 1, 1897)

Again, speaking of Kellogg's contribution to humanitarian and welfare endeavors, White reprimands the Adventist churches in America when stating that the "very work Dr. Kellogg has been managing is the kind of work *the whole of our churches are bound to do under covenant relation to God.* They are to love God supremely and their neighbor as themselves (HM, Nov. 1, 1897).

While White acknowledged that the role of medical institutions was very important to train physicians and nurses for medical missionary roles, her greater emphasis was directed towards all believers, and particularly the clergy, having a capacity to provide simple treatments and remedies in the homes of the communities in which they resided. She envisaged that the medical ministry model would be very broad encompassing a number of vocations as the following selection of quotes indicate:

> Let our *ministers,* who have gained an experience in preaching the word, learn how to give simple treatments and then labor intel-ligently as medical missionary evangelists. (9T: 172)

In every place the sick may be found, and those who go forth as *workers for Christ* should be true health reformers, prepared to give those who are sick the simple treatments that will relieve them, and then pray with them. Thus they will open the door for the entrance of truth. (MM: 320)

All *gospel workers* should know how to give simple treatments that do so much to relieve pain and remove disease. (CH: 389)

As the *canvasser* goes from place to place, he will find many who are sick. He should have a practical knowledge of the causes of disease and should understand how to give simple treatments that he may relieve the suffering ones. (CH: 463)

In the fifty-eighth chapter of Isaiah the Lord tells us plainly what the work is that he requires of us. In order that our *young people* may be fully prepared to do this work, small sanitariums are to be connected with our schools. The students are to be taught how to use nature's simple remedies in the treatment of disease. (RH, Sept. 9, 1902)

God's people are to be genuine medical missionaries. They are to learn to minister to the needs of soul and body. They should know how to give the simple treatments that do so much to relieve pain and remove disease. They should be familiar with the principles of health reform, that they may show others how, by right habits of eating, drinking, and dressing, disease may be prevented and health regained. (WM: 127)

Schwarz, in his introduction to *The Perils of Growth 1886—1905* notes that the trends that had become increasingly apparent in the two decades following official church organisation in 1863 "gained momentum as the nineteenth century waned." The development of educational and health institutions accompanied by an expansion of international mission activities absorbed ever-increasing amounts of Seventh-day Adventist finances and energy. "It was clear by the 1890s that organizational structure was inadequate for the growing church" (1986: 95). Of further concern for Ellen White was the centralization of authority invested in a few men when the needs of the growing church demanded change. White, when addressing a representative group of leaders the day prior to the session opening, pointed out that with the "rapid growth and extension of the work in all the world the responsibilities resting upon the few should be widely distributed"

(Robinson, 1965: 305). Referring to the need for organizational change, including a wider delegation of power, she states:

> Never should the mind of one man or the minds of a few men be regarded as sufficient in wisdom and power to control the work and say what plans shall be followed. The burden of the work in this broad field should not rest upon two or three men. We are not reaching a high standard which, with the great and important truth we are handling, God expects us to reach. (5BIO: 76)

The 1901 General Conference session stands out in SDA history for its emphasis on denominational reorganization in an effort to strengthen various administrative departments

Dr. Kellogg and the Medical Missionary Model

Dr. Kellogg also strongly believed that God's intention for Seventh-day-Adventists was that they would become "medical missionary people," for this type of ministry represented the heart of "true Christianity" (1906: 129, 133). Many Adventists, however, were reluctant to identify wholly with Kellogg's emphasis. George I. Butler, a former General Conference President of the SDA church, articulated the sentiments of many members when communicating with Kellogg:

> It is an excellent thing to heal the sick; encourage the suffering; do good to those who are in great need of help; alleviate pain—that is all good, but my Brother, the salvation of God in his everlasting kingdom, and a preparation for the coming of Christ is more than that. (cited in Wilson, 2014: 57)

Once again, the sectarian tension concerning the prioritization between preaching and teaching doctrine and engaging in Christian humanitarian welfare is abundantly evident.

What is far less obvious, however, is that prior to 1893 contentions between Kellogg and the medical workers on the one hand, and ministerial and administrative employees of the church, on the other, were relatively benign, and a congenial relationship existed between Ellen White and Dr. Kellogg. The tensions and issues that culminated in the final departure of Dr. Kellogg from the SDA church including the severance of the medical work from the ministry in the early twentieth century were the result of a conglomeration of factors that have been well documented over the years and are considered in the following chapter. Suffice to say, that those same issues have subjectively clouded the immense contribution to Adventist health reform, and resonance with Ellen White's three angels' messages emphasis that Kellogg advocated prior to the 1890s. In other words, "the Kellogg of 1893 was a far cry from the Kellogg of a decade or more later" (Fielder, 2012: 99).

Doctrine and Deed

On Friday morning April 3, 1903 at the General Conference meetings, Ellen White, in an address entitled "Our Duty to Leave Battle Creek" reminisced about the impact of John Harvey Kellogg's conversion during the epochal 1888 General Conference in Minneapolis:

> The managers of the Battle Creek Sanitarium have done nobly in the past in regard to trying to maintain a right religious influence in the sanitarium. For a long time there were men connected with the institution whose work it was to hold Bible-readings with the patients, as the way opened Dr. Kellogg fully accorded with this. After the meeting at Minneapolis, Dr. Kellogg was a converted man, and we all knew it. We could see the converting power of God working in his heart and life.

Contextualization is important in any form of research, and to understand the above statement by Ellen White concerning Kellogg's conversion, it must be borne in mind that by 1888, Kellogg had been Medical Director of the Sanitarium for well over a decade. He was well known both within and outside of the denomination and his influence was spreading rapidly. It was not obvious that any outward behavior had been modified by Kellogg; however, the following statement by White may well have been a precipitating factor in his change of heart:

> Grace is unmerited favor, and the believer is justified without any merit of his own, without any claim to offer to God. He is justified through the redemption that is in Christ Jesus, who stands in the courts of heaven as the sinner's substitute and surety. But while he is justified because of the merit of Christ, he is not free to work unrighteousness. Faith works by love and purifies the soul. Faith buds and blossoms and bears a harvest of precious fruit. *Where faith is, good works appear.* The sick are visited, the poor are cared for, the fatherless and the widows are not neglected,

the naked are clothed, the destitute are fed. Christ went about doing good, and when men are united with Him, they love the children of God, and meekness and truth guide their footsteps. (1SM: 398; emphasis supplied)

The implications of this quote seemed to resonate with Kellogg's life-long desire to combine faith with good works; to implement in pragmatic ways SDA theology with humanitarian needs, and this impulse was birthed within eighteen months evidenced by Kellogg's communication with White concerning the need for a church sponsored orphanage.

The year, 1893, for anyone living today appears far too remote to visualize; it was a distant era. Just five years prior, in 1888, one of the greatest theological events in SDA history took place at the annual meeting of the General Conference in Minneapolis, Minnesota. While the outcome of those meetings still produces disagreement within Adventism, they remain a "crucial turning point" in the theological development of the movement (Knight, 1998: 13). Numerous books have been published regarding these meetings; however, Ellen White's summation of the meaning of the 1888 message is encapsulated in the following statement from *Testimonies to Ministers*:

The Lord in His great mercy sent a most precious message to His people through Elders Waggoner and Jones. This message was to bring more prominently before the world the uplifted Saviour, the sacrifice for the sins of the whole world. It presented justification through faith in the Surety; it invited the people to receive the righteousness of Christ, which is made manifest in obedience to all the commandments of God. Many had lost sight of Jesus. They needed to have their eyes directed to His divine person, His merits, and His changeless love for the human family. All power is given into His hands, that He may dispense rich gifts unto men, imparting the priceless gift of His own righteousness to the helpless human agent. This is the message that God commanded to be given to the world. It is the third angel's message, which is to be proclaimed with a loud voice, and attended with the outpouring of His Spirit in a large measure. (1923: 91)

Seventh-day Adventists today may well recall the names Waggoner and Jones, possibly more as a result of their exit from Adventism, rather than their contribution to their church. In 1888, a series of sermons delivered by A. T. Jones concentrated on the theme of the "Third Angel's message." During the 1893 General Conference, the same theme would be elaborated again, however, this time it wasn't by a theologian or minister, rather, a physician.

Dr. Kellogg was scheduled to deliver six lessons concerning the medical missionary work; he actually spoke eight times. Normally, all-important presentations at General Conference Sessions are made available in the pages of the *General Conference Daily Bulletin*. For some reason, perhaps due to developing tensions between Kellogg, the ministry and administration, his presentations were not included. His 'lessons,' which were stenographically recorded, were included, however, in an Extra addition of *The Medical Missionary* magazine published, not by the Review and Herald, a denominational press, but by the Good Health Publishing Company, a Kellogg sponsored paper. Apparently, a lack of funding was the reason provided for the omission of Kellogg's eight presentations in print, yet other less significant issues were included. This scenario led one author to suggest with 'tongue-in-cheek,' that a far more plausible explanation is simply that someone remembered Kellogg's presentation at the previous General Conference session, and saw little value in a repeat discussion concerning 'lard crackers, coiled sausage and 'lively cheese.' Perhaps more to the point was the same author's conclusion that it is "hard to imagine that anything other than an editorial decision decreed that Kellogg would almost entirely disappear from the official record." Perhaps the fact that Kellogg "was a physician rather than a theologian worked against him" (Fielder, 2014: 63).

A brief review of the eight presentations by Kellogg reveals his deep insights into medical missionary work, their relationship to Adventist theology and his understanding of Ellen White. While these insights were neglected and often 'drowned out' by the 'noise' due to the tensions of the latter Kellogg years, they nonetheless provide a lens through which to consider the doctor's early thinking and contributions towards the medical ministry work.

Kellogg's first presentation entitled "Needs and Opportunities for Medical Missionary Work," delivered on February 5 commenced by calling the delegates attention to a comment made by Ellen White in 1891 with reference to 'opening doors' for the gospel:

> How shall the Lord's work be done? How can we gain access to souls buried in midnight darkness? Prejudice must be met; corrupt religion is hard to deal with. The very best ways and means of work must be prayerfully considered. There is a way in which many doors will be opened to the missionary. Let him become

intelligent in the care of the sick, as a nurse, or learn how to treat disease, as a physician; and if he is imbued with the spirit of Christ, what a field of usefulness is opened before him! (*The Medical Missionary*, Extra, No.1, March, 1893: 1; CH, 1923: 33)

Kellogg agreed with White's evaluation and supported the need for both medical missionary work and personnel:

> We want men and women who will become medical missionaries. There are other things that we need, but we need men and women most of all. Medical missionaries are needed in every large city. Sister White says this upon the subject . . . "In every large city there should be not two or three, but scores of well organized, well-disciplined workers." (*The Medical Missionary*, Extra, No.1, March, 1893: 3; MM: 300)

The Gospel of the Third Angel's Message

On February 9, Dr. Kellogg provided his second presentation entitled "The Medical Missionary Himself," which focused on the need for those engaged in God's work to be especially careful to maintain their own health. One suspects, that much of the presentation was primarily intended for the ministry due to Kellogg's growing dismay at the clergy's unfaithfulness to health reform (Fielder, 2014: 67).

> Three or four hours after eating, a dyspeptic often feels giddy, stupid, and sleepy, with a dull headache, and a pressure in the back of the head. He thinks he has worked or studied too hard. That is all nonsense. A man may work every day as hard as he can, and not have the headache, or injure his brain. Few people have brains enough to be hurt by work. I am sure I have not. The trouble is not in the head; it is down below, in the stomach . . . Every portion of his body is saturated with these poisonous matters. (*The Medical Missionary*, Extra, No.1, March, 1893: 10; 3T: 235)

Kellogg then proceeded to direct the discussion towards matters both theological and ministerial:

> Calvinism originated in that kind of body. I have no doubt that the doctrine of everlasting torment originated in the same way, among the monks shut up in cloisters without exercise, until their bodies became saturated with dingy poisons, and they wrote their dingy

theology under these influences. (*The Medical Missionary*, Extra, No.1, March, 1893: 10; 3T: 235)

The doctor then invokes a comment by White concerning the relationship between the mind and body, where she states, "If you would exercise your muscles, your mind would be better balanced, your thoughts would be purer and more elevated, and your sleep would be more natural and healthy." Kellogg quickly picked up on the final statement, "your mind would be better balanced," and left little doubt as to where he took aim, declaring, "Now if there is a man who needs to have his mind better balanced than a minister or a laborer in these institutions, I do not know who he is. Do not we, more than any other class of people on earth, need well balanced minds?" (*The Medical Missionary*, Extra, No.1, March, 1893: 10; 3T: 3, 235).

Finally, Kellogg sought to demonstrate the interconnectedness between the gospel and health reform citing a statement from the pen of White to introduce his point (Fielder, 2014: 69). Of particular significance is Kellogg's choice of quote associating health reform with the third angel's message. "Our preachers should all be genuine, sincere health reformers, not merely adopting the reform because others do, but in obedience to the word of God." The doctor in his own words then proceeds to explain White's counsel. "What does it mean? It means that our preachers should all understand that the word of God says they must be genuine, sincere health reformers, and that they are not obeying God unless they are such." Furthermore, declares Kellogg, "Now when you preach righteousness by faith, don't forget to put health reform in, and then I believe the third angels' message will go with great power. Temperance is a part of the third angel's message." Kellogg concludes, "You can't preach the third angel's message without preaching hygiene and temperance in it. The Lord has put it there to make us better men and women, to save us from fanaticism, to give us health and strength and vigor with which to carry on this important work" (*The Medical Missionary*, Extra, No.1, March, 1893: 11; 3T: 3, 311).

The following day Dr. Kellogg's theme was direct as direct as was it's title: "The Duty of Charity and Benevolence." On this occasion, the Bible, rather than White's writings were cited. Again, he sought to impress upon his hearers that Adventists were to be 'doers' of the Word; not just passive hearers of the Word. Once more, the clergy, the intended recipients of the doctor's comments, were made abundantly obvious in the following comment:

> The Apostle says, in substance, that if one sees another who is suf-
> fering and needy and afflicted, and turns away without ministering
> to his wants, he has not the love of God in him, no matter what
> his profession may be, no matter what splendid sermons he can
> preach, or how zealously he can exhort, or how earnestly he can
> pray; no matter how diligent he may be in distributing tracts; and
> in doing in various ways what he supposes to be 'giving the third
> angel's message;' nevertheless the love of God is not in him. (*The
> Medical Missionary*, Extra, No.1, March, 1893: 11)

Kellogg was annoyed that Christians, including Seventh-day Adventists, were content to cite scripture upon scripture, yet failed in applying
those same biblical utterances in reality. He was more concerned with
biblical *application* then mere sermonizing. The doctor, as an example,
was scathing as he contextualised his thoughts and comments when referring to the lethargic attitude and response towards efforts to provide
for those requiring such care:

> For years and years we have been well able to furnish a Home for
> the aged, the infirm, the homeless; for poor widows, worn-out
> ministers, aged pilgrims, and helpless children, members of our
> denomination, old pioneers in the cause, who gave liberally of
> their property in the early days when the work was just begin-
> ning, and whose faith in the truths which we profess has led them
> to put all their earnings into the cause instead of hoarding up a
> competency for themselves—all these worthy and deserving ones
> who appeal to us on fraternal as well as humanitarian grounds, we
> have neglected in a manner which has become a denominational
> disgrace. (*The Medical Missionary*, Extra, No.1, March, 1893: 11)

While Kellogg was charged in his later years as being unbalanced towards philanthropic and humanitarian work, he was seeking, at this time,
to rectify what he believed was an imbalance towards those in Adventism
proclaiming doctrine without associated deeds. Kellogg was adamant that
one's theology is not a static process but requires action in response. In the
same presentation, he "drove the nail" very close to home concerning his
church's overall lackluster concern for their own flock:

> I have in my possession the positive proof that worthy Seventh-
> day Adventists are left by their brethren and sisters to become a
> public charge, and are today in country poorhouses. Worthy old
> pilgrims, aged men and aged women, have been left to die among
> strangers who had no care or affection for them, deprived of kind

sympathy as well as common comforts. (*The Medical Missionary,* Extra, No.1, March, 1893: 12).

At this point, Kellogg, simultaneously acknowledges SDA irresponsibility in providing care for their own people while brazenly declaring that the supposed eschatological persecutor of the remnant people as being more concerned for the welfare of others, including Adventists, than the remnant are for their own:

> Even Catholic orphan asylums have been opened to receive Seventh-day Adventist orphans. Yet we claim to be a 'peculiar' people.' Is it not about time we began to be 'zealous of good works?' (*The Medical Missionary,* Extra, No.1, March, 1893: 12)

Dr. Kellogg was seeking to challenge a misconception held by many within Adventism that theology was all that mattered, and as such, the medical missionary work was deemed unconnected with Adventism's rationale for existence—preaching the third angel's message:

> You will easily remember the time when medical missionary was first talked about, and also that everybody looked askance at it, because, as they thought, it was something foreign to our work. The idea seemed to prevail that we had a special work to spread the third angel's message, and that the Lord did not want our attention to be diverted into foreign channels. For some years I have been studying the Bible with special reference to this subject, and it seems to me that what we call humanitarian work, or medical missionary work, is just as much a part of the third angel's message as any other work connected with it; certainly no one connected with the third angel's message ought to be any the less a Christian than members of other denominations. (*The Medical Missionary,* Extra, No.1, March, 1893: 13)

It is apparent that Kellogg was not reluctant nor shy in pointing out the deficiencies in his church and sought to remind church members in general, and the ministers, in particular, to take the medical missionary work seriously. His comments, while at times, quite abrasive, were nonetheless reckoned, by the doctor, to be accurate.

In one of his final presentations, Kellogg referred to Matthew 25: 31–46, the parable of the sheep and the goats with which all Adventists were very familiar. No Adventist could have left the meeting in a state of ambiguity regarding Kellogg's assessment that practical Christianity was a determining factor in the judgement:

> Now who are the "righteous"? Why, the righteous are those that did clothe the naked, and did visit the sick, and did feed the hungry, and gave drink to the thirsty. They are the righteous. Now, does not this state as strongly as possible that the Lord wants us to do these things, and that we are not righteous unless we do them? No matter how much faith we profess, unless we have done these things, we are not righteous at all. When we come up in the Judgment, the test question will not be, "Did you preach the third angel's message? Did you give Bible-readings?" but, "Did you feed the hungry, clothe the naked?" etc., because these are fundamental things, while the other things are matters which naturally grow out of doing these fundamental things. (*The Medical Missionary*, Extra, No.1, March, 1893: 17)

Dr. Kellogg was irritated that with so much instruction, from both the Bible and Ellen White, why the Adventists church as a whole, couldn't or perhaps wouldn't just admit that the medical missionary endeavor, is fundamentally, the Lord's work. Speaking of the need for 'good works,' Kellogg cited a selection of White's comments commencing in 1859 through 1876, in his daily presentations. "One reason people look down upon us," the doctor declared, "is, that they never heard that Seventh-day Adventists have ever done anything in the way of benevolence." He continues by asking, "Did the world ever hear of us as a people especially interested in the welfare of the widow, the orphan, the afflicted, and the needy?" Concluding, he answers his own question, "We have no reputation of that kind in the world. . . ." Kellogg then reflects on the past concerning the lackluster response to Ellen White's counsel:

> We had a testimony over thirty years ago, saying that we as a special people were to "rise higher and higher," but it does not appear, from testimonies received at different times since that one was given, that we have risen perceptibly from that time until now—a period of over thirty years. . . . We must do the work which the Lord has told us to do, and which we have left undone. We must do our duty in relation to health principles and benevolence in connection with other questions (*The Medical Missionary*, Extra, No.1, March, 1893: 28–29).

White, in 1900, once again stated the need for combining doctrine with deed; precept with practice:

> As we near the close of time, we must rise higher and still higher on the question of health reform and Christian temperance,

presenting it in a more positive and decided manner. We must strive continually to educate the people, not only by our words but by our practice. Precept and practice combined have a telling influence. (CD: 443)

The remainder of Kellogg's presentations elaborated on the two main causes established in the first few days at the 1893 General Conference session: the adoption of health reform principles and Christian benevolence, both of which, he believed, were unquestionably supported by the Bible and Ellen White, and were fundamental to finishing God's work in the context of the third angel's message (Fiedler, 2014: 101).

The relationship between Kellogg, on the one hand, and White, the clergy, and church administrators, on the other, witnessed occasional and at times intense disagreements up until the mid-1890s. From the late 1890s through to the 1907 when Dr. Kellogg's church membership was revoked, however, a transition towards total estrangement became increasingly evident, the impact of which continues to reverberate within Adventism. It would be naïve to suggest that the issues culminating in Dr. Kellogg's departure from Adventist were singular and simplistic. The evidence of historical research indicates otherwise and suggests that a closer investigation reveals multiple issues and circumstances came into play over time that pushed 'erring mortals on both sides of the conflict to the point of rupture" (Fiedler, 2014: 119). It is towards an understanding of those processes that the following chapter is concerned.

6

Tensions in a Maturing Millennialist Movement

In the *American Journal of Health Promotion*, the editor, Michael O'Donnell describes health promotion as the science and art of assisting people change their lifestyle towards a state of optimal health. Optimal health is defined as a balance of emotional, physical, social, spiritual and intellectual health (Nieman, 1992: 123). If Ellen White had the greatest influence on the consciousness of Adventists, on the basis of her prophetic utterances, in many respects, Dr. J. H. Kellogg was Adventism's social gospel advocate (Plantak, 1998: 59). There can be little doubt that Kellogg's contribution towards changing the lifestyle habits of the American population was both profound and arguably unsurpassed (Willis, 2003: 99).

Former US Labor Minister, Senator James J. Davis, wrote of Kellogg, in the *Battle Creek Enquirer and News* on December 15, 1943 following Kellogg's death, "His was a life rich with service—a life dedicated to the improvement of science of nutrition and the science of human health." In the same article, former US President Herbert Hoover added the following remarks: "Dr Kellogg has lived a long and exceedingly useful life. Many thousands owe their health and happiness to him" (Willis, 2003: 96). It is of no small interest that while Kellogg's enormous impact on the health of the American public was far greater than White's, he was one of few Adventists at the time to take her views on health seriously (Bull & Lockhart, 2007: 302).

The Battle for the Essential Frame of Reference

Knight (1998: 142) argues that the essential difference between White and the reformers of her day, including Kellogg, was philosophical. That is, every subject she dealt with she handled within the *great controversy frame of reference*, or the galactic struggle between Christ and Satan. More specifically, as noted in chapter 4, she set forth her counsel for both daily living and reform in the context of the three angel's messages of Revelation 14: 6–12, which includes Adventism's mission to a troubled world facing the imminent premillennial return of Christ to earth (emphasis supplied).

Plantak asserts that there was no doubt in White's mind that evangelism is the primary task of the church, and that the Seventh-day Adventist movement was birthed to proclaim a particular message including Sabbath observance, judgement, and the impending Second Advent of Christ (1998: 55). Having said such, White, at times, went beyond narrow exclusiveness by outlining the duty of the Seventh-day Adventists in service to the poor and oppressed in three distinct lines: 1) the church community or local congregation, 2) the local community, and 3) the world community (Plantak, 1998: 54).

Adventists are compelled, White believed, to help the less fortunate brothers and sisters as did the early New Testament community (Acts 2: 44–46). Furthermore, this service must be provided to others, "irrespective of their faith." She continues by declaring that the work of supporting the needy, the suffering, the oppressed, and the destitute, is the self-same work, which every church should long have since been doing. "We are to show the tender sympathy of the Samaritan in supplying physical necessities, feeding the hungry, bringing the poor that are cast out to our homes, gathering from God every day grace and strength that will enable us to reach the very depths of human misery and help those who cannot help themselves" (6T: 276). White did not downgrade toil for the needy to a secondary function of the gospel, however, the core of the gospel, for her, remained human restoration, and the work of the gospel included sharing both spiritual and temporal benefits (Rock, 1988: 6).

Clearly, both White and Kellogg considered health reform as a vital element to the betterment of humankind and as part of the salvation process, however, by the late 1890s, the foundations from which those reforms emanated were fundamentally different. Bull and Lockhart summarize those differences well when arguing that for Kellogg, what mattered most was not one's theology, but one's state of health. His overriding concern, which was the essence of biological living, was making sick people better and keeping them well when they attained good health. Continuing, the same authors declare that White also considered health reform to be a crucial component in the salvation process, but for her it was an adjunct to, or an attachment, rather than the foundation of the Adventist health message (2007: 303). Thus, good health was a central factor in the betterment of humankind for both individuals, however, Kellogg remained adamant that commitment to the religion of biological living should not be constrained by theological limitations; White, on the other hand, maintained that health reform must remain secondary to primary theological principles.

While the ultimate direction that health reform in Adventism would take at the commencement of the twentieth century resulted largely in a power struggle between Kellogg and his church over a number of issues, the core concern lay far deeper than a difference in personal opinions; they actually centered on the future direction of Seventh-day Adventist thought, practice and ongoing identity (Douglass, 1998: 294). It is to these issues that we now address.

Health Reform and SDA identity: Arm or Body?

In the *Review and Herald*, November 8, 1870 edition, James White recalls a vision received in the autumn of 1848, four years following the Great Disappointment, in which his wife, Ellen, was shown the harmful effects of tobacco use and the consumption of tea and coffee. An enquiring man in 1851 seeking clarification inquired of Ellen White whether she had actually seen in 'vision' that it was "wrong to use tobacco." White's response was both swift and direct stating, "I have seen in vision that tobacco was a filthy weed, and that it must be laid aside or given up." She elaborates further suggesting that Jesus seeks to perfect His children when declaring, "I saw that Christ will have a church without spot or wrinkle or any such thing to present to His Father, . . . as He leads us through the pearly gates of the New Jerusalem. . . . We must be perfect Christians, deny ourselves all the way along, tread the narrow, thorny pathway that our Jesus trod, and then if we are final overcomers, heaven, sweet heaven will be cheap enough" (1Bio: 224).

Fifteen years later in June 1863, when White received her major health vision, among the several health principles enunciated, a new emphasis was detected: the relationship between "physical welfare and spiritual health, or holiness" (Robinson, 1965: 77). "I saw that it was a sacred duty," wrote Write, "to attend to our health, and arouse others to their duty. ... We have a duty to speak out against intemperance of every kind. ..." In the same letter, she also wrote, "the work God requires of us will not shut us away from caring for our health. The more perfect our health, the more perfect will be our labor" (3SM: 280).

A further health vision in Rochester, New York on Christmas day, 1865 was given White in which she states that "I was shown that our Sabbathkeeping people have been negligent in acting upon the light which God has given in regard to health reform; that there is yet a great work before us; and that, as a people, we have been too backward in God's opening providence, as He has chosen to lead us" (1T: 485, 486).

What is of interest is that the first health reform vision given to White in 1863 outlined the major health principles and urged their adoption by the Adventist believers, while the second vision pointed out that the response to God's leading was underwhelming, to say the least. Of even more significance, however, is that for the first time, White connects health reform within the context of preparation for Christ's soon Advent as depicted in the third angel's message of Revelation 14. "The health reform, I was shown, is a part of the third angel's message and is just as closely connected with it as are the arm and hand with the human body. I saw that we as a people must make an advance move in this great work. Ministers and people must act in concert" (1T: 486–488).

From this point onwards, White consistently linked health reform with what she perceived was Adventism's raison d'être—proclamation of and preparation for, the imminent return of Christ. Douglass suggests that the linking of health reform and the everlasting gospel was based on three principles:

1. *The Humanitarian principle.* Both by example and teaching, White consistently emphasized that the "work of health reform is the Lord's means for lessening suffering in our world . . . ." (3T: 62; 9T: 112).

2. *The Evangelical principle.* Health reform is to a bridge or conduit by which the gospel can meet people where they are. This is why White, in the context of medical missionary work, stated that the health message "is the pioneer work of the gospel, the door through which the truth for this time is to find entrance to many homes. . . . A demonstration of the principles of health reform will do much toward removing prejudice against our evangelical work. The Great Physician, the originator of medical missionary work, will bless all who thus seek to impart the truth for this time" (Ev: 513, 514). Specifically concerning Adventist health institutions, she wrote: "God desires our health institutions to stand as witnesses for the truth" (MM: 187). Furthermore, the rationale for receiving unbelievers into sanitariums "is to lead them to embrace truth (1T: 560).

3. *The Soteriological principle.* To ready a people, both physically and spiritually for the Second Advent was the distinctive tenant of Adventist health reform in the nineteenth century. "He who cherishes the light which God has given him upon health reform has an important aid in the work of becoming sanctified through the truth, and fitted for immortality" (CD: 15, 59–60). Thus, the primary purpose that distinguished White's health reform agenda was to join the spiritual and the physical in a wholistic union on the practical, day-to-day experience of the average person (Douglass, 1998: 291–292).

Institutional Growth Priorities

At the turn of the twentieth century, Adventism was struggling with the enormous growing strength of the 'right arm.' Estimates suggest that in 1901 Kellogg's Medical Missionary and Benevolent Association employed around 2,000 workers compared to 1,500 employed by the General Conference of Seventh-day Adventists. Kellogg's abundant energy, facile pen, creative imagination, and administrative prowess, made him by 1900 arguably the most well known SDA on earth (Schwarz, 1979: 278–283).

Financial and managerial issues have been a constant threat to the survival and mission of Adventist health institutions since the opening of the Western Health Reform Institute in 1866, which is a classic example. No sooner had the Institute opened its doors to customers, the call to enlarge its facilities by the medical superintendent was made because they feared they would not be able to accommodate adequately those that may wish to come. The Institute's three original buildings were fully occupied and available rooms in neighbouring homes were sought to rectify the matter. The proposal to build another *large* building to rectify the matter was imperative, the administrator argued (RH, Jan. 8, 1867). In *The Health Reformer* of March 1867, Dr. Lay spoke of the difficulty in finding rooms to accommodate the daily arrival of new patients. "We would say," declared Lay "that we hope the time is not far distant when we shall have room enough to accommodate two or three hundred patients. Perhaps this will be no further distant than next autumn. We trust every true friend of the cause will continue to work with ardor and zeal." $15,000 was required immediately to complete the newly proposed building and readers of the *Review and Herald* were notified accordingly. The writers of the *Review and Herald* articles cited statements from the pen of Ellen White to support their soliciting endeavors. Interestingly, no further mention was made in either the *Review and Herald* or *The Health Reformer* after the first appeal for financial assistance. The reason, however, soon became obvious.

Both Ellen and James White had been unable to attend the annual meeting of the Health Reform Institute, primarily on the basis of James's poor health, however, it was with serious trepidation that they heard of the plans to greatly enlarge the infant institution (Robinson, 1965: 175). Ellen shared her feelings towards the planned developments, proclaiming that the "disposition manifested to crowd the matter of the institute so fast has been one of the heaviest trials I have ever borne" (1T: 563). She wrote to the directors of the institute, declaring that the plans presented to her in vision revealed that the Health Reform Institute should be small at the beginning, and guardedly increased, as good physicians and staff could be acquired and means raised as the wants of the sick should demand. Furthermore, White gave voice to her concerns about the hefty calculations being hastily urged by the administrators. She was also quick to remind the directors not to dismiss the fact, that many of the hygienic institutions started in the United States within the last twenty-five years, but few maintain even a visible existence at the present time" (1T: 558, 559).

White's concern was one of priorities, that is, in their enthusiasm over the health reform movement a number of the brethren were in danger of giving it a position of unwarranted importance. She requested that the Health Institute be allowed to grow, as all the other interests among us have grown, but only as fast as it can do so safely without crippling the other branches of the Adventist work, which are of equal or greater importance. (1T: 559, 560).

The major danger, in White's estimation, was placing undue attention and means on health reform at the expense of other branches of the mission of the church. Particularly, galling to her was institutional debt, which placed in jeopardy other important avenues of church mission. Referring to the need to prioritize, she again reiterated that while health reform is intimately connected with the Adventism's eschatological message, it is not the message. "Our preachers should teach the health reform, yet they should not make this the leading theme in the place of the message," she declared. Furthermore, as a people, "we should take hold of every reform with zeal, yet should avoid giving the impression that we are vacillating and subject to fanaticism" (1T: 559).

On another occasion, and in similar, consistent tones, White elaborated on the connection between preaching and health principles. She made it abundantly clear that that health reform cannot usurp the place of preaching, in particular, proclaiming Revelation 14, the commandments of God and the testimony of Jesus, for White was adamant this this is the burden of our work. The "presentation of health principles must be united with this message, but must not in any case be independent of it, or in any way take the place of it"(CD: 75). During the next several decades, White was found to be 'beating the same drum' concerning SDA health institutions.

Issues related to the rebuilding of the Battle Creek Sanitarium following its destruction by fire on February 18, 1902 epitomize the growing tensions between White and Kellogg. At the time of the fire, Kellogg was returning to Battle Creek by train from the West Coast and first heard of the news on arrival in Chicago. Undeterred, as the train continued its journey towards Battle Creek, he called into action his entrepreneurial skills, requesting a table and utilized the remaining two hours in drawing up plans for the new Sanitarium (A. L. White, 1981: 150). White felt a pressing need to communicate with Kellogg as to the future plans and development of the Battle Creek enterprise, emphasizing two points, in particular: the desirability of "smaller sanitariums" be built in a range of locations and the temptation facing Kellogg to "build up a very great work that would glorify him with a fruitage for which the sanitarium is established, but in reverse to the sanitarium's size (A. L. White, 1981: 150).

Kellogg quickly abandoned any thought of relocating and one week after the destruction of the institution, he published in the *Review and Herald* his dream for Battle Creek, envisioning a new, fireproof building, bigger and better than the previous structure. It was to be an edifice "standing as a temple of truth, the headquarters for a worldwide movement, represented by hundreds of physicians and nurses, and many thousands of interested friends in all parts of the world" (RH, Feb. 25, 1902).

White was distressed and her fundamental concerns regarding the continuing imbalance of the 'arm with the body' is evident in a letter written to Kellogg in April, 1902 stating that she had been given a message specifically for the Doctor. She elaborates, declaring, "you have had many cautions and warnings, which I sincerely hope and pray you will consider." White continues to reprimand Kellogg maintaining that she was instructed to, "tell you that the great display you are making in Battle Creek is not after God's order. You are planning to build in Battle Creek a larger sanitarium than should be erected there." White was concerned that Kellogg's new plans of centralization would place an enormous drain on the church's finances and function. "There are other parts of the Lord's vineyard in which buildings are greatly needed," she avowed, and Battle Creek is not to be made a New Jerusalem. "Do not erect in immense institution in Battle Creek which will make it necessary for you to draw upon our people for means," she cautioned for such a "building might far better be divided, and plants made in many places. Over and over again this has been presented to me" (Letter, 125, 1902). While the centralization of Adventist institutions in Battle Creek, including the desire to construct a larger sanitarium caused great concern and anxiety for White, the identity and ethos of the Battle Creek sanitarium was even more disturbing.

Adventist Health Institutions—a Question of Identity

In the course of his long arduous campaign to promote biological living in an attempt to convert Americans to a healthier lifestyle, Kellogg utilized a wide variety of means including the written page, public speaking engagements, personal communication with friends and peers etc. The most effective means, however, involved his leadership of the Battle Creek sanitarium. He reluctantly agreed to serve for one year as the sanitarium's chief physician; history records that he remained connected in various capacities with the institution for 67 years (Schwarz, 2006: 62).

During the recharting of the Battle Creek Sanitarium in the late 1890s the enunciation of the terms, "undenominational and unsectarian" first appeared (Schwarz, 1979: 284). The seeds of change first appeared in 1893, however, when Kellogg began to insist that the medical work conducted by Seventh-day Adventists was a "great Christian benevolent work, not particularly denominational in character" (A. L. White, 1981: 160). It was during this time that the Seventh-day Adventist Medical Missionary and Benevolent Association formed to replace the former Health and Temperance Association. A further three years later in 1896, a name change occurred resulting in the words 'Seventh-day Adventist' being replaced with 'International.' Dr Kellogg insisted that the purpose of the organisation was to "carry forward medical and philanthropic independent of any sectarian or denominational control, in home and foreign lands." The following year at a convention of the association it was declared that the delegates in attendance were "here as Christians" and not "as Seventh-day Adventists (A. L. White, 1981: 160). Nor were they in attendance for the purpose of presenting or supporting anything "that is peculiarly Seventh-day Adventist in doctrine" (Wilson, 2014: 58).

Although the Battle Creek sanitarium was founded as an SDA institution, the original charter expired in 1897. Kellogg was entrusted by the sanitarium directors with the task of securing a new charter, required by the Michigan State, resulting in the formation a new Michigan Sanitarium and Benevolent Association that would acquire the assets and continue to maintain the work of the Western Health Reform Institute. Kellogg was particularly anxious that the sanitarium be legally recognized as a charitable organisation. As part of the requirements of the new Association, members were required to sign a declaration of principles, which included a statement approving the non-profit rationale of the Association and agreeing that the sanitarium's function would be of an unsectarian, undenominational, humanitarian and philanthropic nature (Schwarz, 1979: 284).

When a number of prospective members of the new Association expressed concerns about the use of the wording, 'undenominational' and 'unsectarian,' Kellogg, sought to disarm their fears stating that there was no issue at all and that the words meant simply that the sanitarium was "to be conducted as a medical institution, that it may have the advantages of the statutes of the state; as a hospital, it must be carried on as an undenominational institution. It cannot give benefits to a certain class, but must be for the benefit of any who are sick." Furthermore, the "institution may support any work it chooses with the earnings of the Association, but cannot discriminate against anyone because of his beliefs" (Schwarz, 1979: 284). The Association members readily accepted Kellogg's explanation.

The growing number of declarations made by Dr. Kellogg and associates supporting the non-denominational and non-sectarian status of the Battle Creek sanitarium evoked considerable alarm within the Adventist ranks. In midsummer of 1902, White responded unequivocally. "It has been stated that the Battle Creek Sanitarium is not denominational," she argued, "but if ever an institution was established to be denominational in every sense of the word, this sanitarium was." White then proceeds with a rationale for the existence of health reform institutions. "Why are sanitariums established if it is not that they may be the right hand of the gospel in calling the attention of men and women to the truth that we are living amid the perils of the last days?" And yet, in one sense, it remains true that the Sanitarium is undenominational, but only in that it receives "as patients peoples of all classes and all denominations" (SHM: 253).

The difference of interpretation concerning between White and Kellogg concerning the word 'undenominational' is blatantly stark. White had earlier indicated that the original Western Health Reform Institute be operated in a non-sectarian manner in terms of accepting clientele, but under no circumstances was this to insinuate a diminution of the institution Adventist roots and heritage. Nor, nor did she see the point of Seventh-day Adventist missions that did not in some way promote Adventism's eschatological message (Wilson, 2014: 58). Kellogg was equally determined and as adamant that SDA theological distinctives should not hinder humanitarian efforts. When Kellogg stated that the sanitarium was not in the business of presenting anything peculiarly Adventist in doctrine he was in reality placing the sanitarium on a course that diverged from traditional Adventism. That is, the "institution met the outside world on medical and humanitarian grounds rather than on a specifically Adventist basis." Again, one's state of health was a priority for Kellogg, even if it trumped one's theology (Bull & Lockhart, 2007: 303). This perspective was clearly discernible in Kellogg's approach to benevolent humanitarianism and welfare work.

The Social Gospel and Non-Sectarian Adventism

As a skillful promoter, Kellogg had convinced the General Conference leadership in 1893 to organize the Medical Missionary and Benevolent Association, whose purpose was to coordinate and direct all Adventist health facilities, including social service organizations, orphanages and homes for the aged. With Kellogg as its president, the association began to encourage the development of welfare-based missions in cities across America. The anticipated financing of these endeavors from Adventist health institutions and at times solicitation from Adventist members proved woefully inadequate resulting in Kellogg seeking other means of financial revenue, including the public purse. Forced to turn to the public for ongoing contributions, Kellogg began to emphasize the non-sectarian orientation of the missions.

As 1899 dawned, it had becoming abundantly obvious that Kellogg was taking steps to divest the medical missionary work from "its denominational ties, in the Battle Creek Sanitarium, the medical school, and in the work for the outcasts and socially deprived classes in Chicago" (A. L. White, 1983: 394). His uncompromising zealousness for biological living often placed him in a precarious position with Adventist leaders. He consistently maintained that SDAs should focus exclusively on being medical missionaries throughout the world, for this work was the heart of 'true Christianity' and in the final judgement one's participation in the medical missionary work, would comprise the ultimate test—not one's biblical astuteness (Wilson, 2014: 56). "The world is dying and if ever there was a need of live, earnest, medical missionaries, it is now," Kellogg insisted. "If there ever was a time when the medical missionary element of the gospel should appear in its proper place on an equal footing with the preaching of the kingdom as in the commission given by Christ to his disciples, now is the time" (Kellogg, 1906: 129–133).

Dr. Kellogg sincerely believed that humanitarian work would accomplish better results in winning converts to Adventism than all the SDA ministers combined (Schwarz, 1964: 335, 338). The pragmatics of this ideology witnessed the establishment of sanitariums in the USA and the denomination's first orphanage in 1891. In 1893, he became the first director of the Seventh-day Adventist Medical Missionary and Benevolent Association (MMBA), which controlled the denomination's humanitarian work. It was through this organisation that Kellogg primarily ministered to society's outcasts, disadvantaged, poor, and the unemployed" (Bull and Lockhart, 2007: 304).

Kellogg advocated a social gospel that differed significantly for mainstream Adventism; it was a gospel void of sectarian trammels (Schwarz, 1964: 312). He perceived his church to be a benevolent organisation and that it was significantly more important for a person to be a good

Samaritan than to be a good theologian (Schwarz, 1964: 296). Thus, he was particularly concerned to witness his fellow Adventists commit themselves to a broad humanitarian program (Schwarz, 1964: 162). Too many of his fellow church members, insisted Kellogg, held undesirable theories of religion, which consisted primarily of a list mentality, that is, the 'things one can and cannot do' and this type of thinking disempowered an individual from fully engaging in humanitarian programs.

The doctor's personal financial support and resourcing of humanitarian endeavors is unquestionable, and he sought to convince Adventist administrators and members to commit to the same financial liberality. An enduring source of tension for Kellogg and the church was, however, that the doctor's financial resources were never adequate to cater for all the charitable projects his mind conceived (Schwarz, 2006: 162). Although Kellogg and SDA church administrators differed in opinion as to the scale of welfare work, this was not the major reason for their split, argues Plantak. The significant issue emerged in their understanding as to the purpose of concern for the poor. The nature of true welfare as far as Kellogg was concerned "was purely to help the poor out of Christian love." Therefore, the welfare work Kellogg envisaged and engaged in had to remain non-sectarian and non-denominational (1998: 64). Kellogg was adamant that when a person helps their neighbor they do it as a Christian, and not as a Baptist, Methodist or a Seventh-day Adventist; SDA leaders believed precisely the opposite, that is, the ultimate goal of welfare activity was to convert people to Adventism (Plantak, 1998: 64).

During the 1890s the United States staggered under one of the most severe financial depressions in its history, yet the same decade witnessed tremendous institutional expansion within Adventism (Schwarz, 1986: 119). Two new colleges had commenced (Union College and Walla Walla). Kellogg was very proactive in the establishment of several medical institutions in the United States and one in Mexico, the first medical facility of the church established outside of America. For all of these institutional endeavors, funds for the capital investments were borrowed and then the General Conference Association was persuaded to undertake the obligations (A. L. White, 1981: 155). As previously noted, debates and disagreements over financial policies to support Adventist health institutions and initiatives were a constant source of conflict between Kellogg and church administrators.

Kellogg was a forceful, persuasive, energetic and at times, intimidating character, to the extent that the General Conference leaders during the 1880s found it increasingly difficult to counter his insistence for financial support and heavy debts were assumed by the church without a systematic plan for their amortization (A. L. White, 1981: 155, 156). This scenario was patently obvious when the Battle Creek Sanitarium was destroyed by fire. Even though the Sanitarium had been operating for thirty-five years, outstanding debts totaled $250,000. Despite good patronage, almost all SDA health institutions struggled under great financial burden, largely due to grandiose building schemes and poor business management. When A. G. Daniells assumed responsibilities as General Conference President in 1901, he was aghast to find that institutional indebtedness was close to $500,000, which in the context of the times represented a huge debt. Records indicate that the top pay for physicians, ministers and publishing house employees at the time was approximately $12 to $15 per week (A. L. White, 1981: 156).

Arguably, none of Kellogg's projects absorbed more finances or served as an example of non-sectarian aid than the Chicago Medical Mission (CMM) opened in 1983. Prior to making a final decision as to the location of the CMM Kellogg visited the Chicago Police Station and requested he be directed to the "dirtiest and wickedest" part of the city. Kellogg insists that his desire to assist those in poverty, and slums was not a natural instinct; rather, he felt a great "physical repugnance" toward the dirty and often drunken slum dwellers and, furthermore, the idea of working with these kind of people had been "terribly disagreeable" for him (Schwarz, 2006: 168). The CMM initially provided three types of aid: a medical dispensary, free laundry and free baths. The character of the mission's neighborhood is evident from the dispensary reports, which indicated that 25–30 knife wounds were treated daily. Two weeks after the CMM opened its doors for treatment, Kellogg reported that an average of 100 persons per day utilized the facilities. After nine months of operation, the mission records indicate that in a single month the facility provided 2,116 baths, 869 other treatments, free laundry for 1,725 people, dressed 427 wounds, gave away 53 drug prescriptions, 31 packages of food and 2,942 articles of clothing (Schwarz, 2006: 170, 171). Four years after the CMM opened its doors to the public, Kellogg reported that more than 200,000 persons had made use of the free laundry services and 75,000 of them had acquired new clothing because of church member's gifts. Schwarz declares that as a result of Kellogg's humanitarian emphasis, his work in Chicago can be seen as the origin of modern Adventist welfare activities (Schwarz, 1969: 20).

The basement of the CMM housed the facilities for both the free baths and the laundry, which some mission workers deemed unnecessary accessories or optional extras. "If the gospel were preached," they maintained, "it would lead men to clean up of their own accord." Kellogg's thesis, however, was fundamentally different: "if the men were cleaned up first, they would be easier to reach with Christian teachings." A mission director of a similar institution told Kellogg, "The moral atmosphere of this community has visibly brightened within the last few days, and it is improving every day, as a result of the influence of your practical presentation of the *gospel of cleanliness*" (Schwarz, 1969: 19).

It is also of interest that Kellogg, in keeping with his non-sectarian policy arranged for an interdenominational committee, under the chairmanship of S. S. Sherin, a Methodist minister, to serve in an advisory capacity to the CMM. These undenominational aspects of the mission, which Kellogg insisted, led to misunderstanding and alienation within the Adventist community, ultimately resulting in the termination of the CMM. In 1898, Kellogg prepared a handbook providing instruction on the operation of city medical missions. In the book he stressed that "the sole object of the medical mission, as well as of other missions, is the salvation of men, but here the intimate relation of mind and body, of health and morals, is recognized as an important factor requiring careful attention and consideration" (1898: 5). As noted on previous occasions, Kellogg stated that the mission is a place to emphasize the saving power of Christ, not to teach theology, and furthermore, denominational activities were secondary and to be kept in the background (1898: 7–20).

Most SDAs were convinced that the only rationale for the existence of the CMM and other similar projects was to proclaim distinctively Adventist religious principles, and they questioned the value of a program that appeared to be increasing and absorbing both the denomination's financial resources and its potential leaders without simultaneously promulgating Adventist beliefs (Schwarz, 2006: 175). Winton Beaven concurs arguing that while a number of issues were obvious between Kellogg, White, and church administrators including the autonomy of the medical work, no-debt policy and the evangelistic role of SDA sanitariums, of even greater conflict was his non-sectarian attitude in supporting general humanitarian service rather than specific Adventist evangelism (1994: 166). The doctor's humanitarianism contributed to the popularity of the health and mission institutions, but in doing so alienated the majority of the leadership in the SDA church. Numbers (2008: 249, 250) declares that Kellogg, as early as 1893, had spoken out against the feeling by some Adventists that the work for the suffering and needy unless done with direct proselytizing motives was of no value in assisting the Adventist cause.

During 1898, White penned seventeen letters to J. H. Kellogg, aggregating some 113 pages; the majority were occasions of caution, while in 1899 a further 26 letters were written (A. L. White, 1983: 397). White initially approved of the doctor's commitment to provide aid to the deprived, drunkards, prostitutes and outcasts in Chicago, but by the end of 1898 she revealed her thoughts on the supposed disproportionate and imbalanced emphasis on social welfare work declaring that while a constant work is to be done for the outcasts, this work is not to be made all-absorbing, because these people will always be with us. "All the means must not be bound up in this work, for the highways have not yet received the message." White concludes by suggesting that there is still a work in the Lord's vineyard to be completed, and that "no one should now visit our churches, and claim from them means to sustain the work of rescuing outcasts. The means to sustain that work should come . . . from those not of our faith (4Bio: 397).

White often withheld from mailing her personal letters to Kellogg, for she sensed that her messages of counsel were not accomplishing what they should, and she wrestled to find a means to protect Kellogg from his unbalanced ways. At the 1899 General Conference session, a letter from White, sent from Australia and entitled "The Work for This Time," was read to the assembled delegates. Referring in particular to Kellogg's apparent misunderstanding of the objectives of the medical missionary work, the letter opened with the following words.

> We are standing on the threshold of great and solemn events. Prophecies are fulfilling. The last great conflict will be short, but terrible. Old controversies will be revived. New controversies will arise. The last warnings must be given to the world. There is a special power in the presentation of truth at the present time; but how long will it continue? Only a little while. If ever there was a crisis, it is now (3SM: 419).

In the same letter White noted that "there is a tendency to make some one line all-absorbing; that which should have the first place becomes a secondary consideration" (A. L. White, 1983: 401). White then addressed the central issue stating that while a great work is being conducted for the uplifting of the fallen and degraded there "is a danger of loading down everyone with this class of work, because of the intensity with which it is carried on. There is danger of leading men to center their energies in this line, when God has called them to another work" (4Bio: 401).

Kellogg's social welfare aspirations and activities alone did not precipitate his eventual break with Adventism, but nonetheless, they played an important part. Church leaders, including White, became increasingly convinced and somewhat skeptical that whilst his work was commendable, it did not promote SDA distinctive doctrinal truths to the world. Richard Schwarz's assessment of the differing trajectories between White and Kellogg's understanding of the purpose for Seventh-day Adventists as portrayed in *Adventism in America* is insightful:

> Although Mrs. White had always supported the work for the poor, sick, and unfortunate, she was concerned because the mission activities that Kellogg was promoting placed a disproportionate emphasis on this line of endeavor. She recognized that many other Christian and non-Christian groups would carry on welfare programs. But these groups were not interested in promoting the Adventist doctrine of an imminent return of Jesus and the need to prepare people who loved him well enough to keep all his commandments, including the Seventh-day Sabbath. Thus she called for a return to the original evangelistic kind of mission (1986: 111).

For his part, Kellogg sensed that denominational emphasis on points of difference with other Christians was redundant; the most important objective was to follow the work of Jesus in aiding the destitute, healing the sick, and teaching the uninformed (Schwarz, 1969: 26).

The Pantheism Crisis

'Pantheism' is derived from two Greek words—*pan*, "all," and *theos*, "God." As such, Douglass observes, "everything manifests the presence of God; nature and God are identical" (1998: 200). During the 1840s and 1850s, one of the ex-Millerite groups named the 'spiritualizers' maintained that Christ had indeed returned in 1844; not literally in person but 'in spirit' to his believers. The issue of conjecture was the emphasis on the reduction of Jesus to that of a 'spirit' rather than a literal, material being. When Kellogg's publication, *The Living Temple* became the conduit for pantheistic ideas to be expressed later in the nineteenth century, White recognized distinct similarities with the 'spiritualizers' that she and husband James had confronted following the Great Disappointment. As a teenager, White declared, "I had to bear testimony against them [sentiments regarding God such as those found in *The Living Temple*] before large companies" (Letter 217, 1903, cited in 5BIO: 304). Prior to the death of James White in 1881, Kellogg had shared his emerging views of God with the Whites and Ellen remembered well that she had confronted them before and warned Kellogg that such theories should never be taught in SDA institutions (Manuscript 70, 1905, cited in 5BIO: 281). *The Living Temple*, published in 1903 contained relatively few concepts that Kellogg had not expressed in one way or another during the 1890s. Whilst the majority of its 568 pages are dedicated to rudimentary discussions of human physiology and the cure of disease, theology permeates the volume and gives it a distinctly religious feel (Wilson, 2014: 85).

By 1897, Kellogg was sharing his pantheistic concepts at a ministerial institute prior to the General Conference session. His presentations were for the most part received with acclaim. Perhaps both ignorance and naiveté prevented individuals from recognizing the underlying themes in statements such as, "What a wonderful thought that this mighty God that keeps the whole universe in order, is in us! . . . What an amazing thing that this almighty, all-powerful, and all-wise God should make Himself a servant of man by giving man a free will—power to direct the energy within his body" (*GCDB*, 1897: 83).

Chapter 3 has dealt in reasonable depth with Kellogg's religion of biological living, including his emphasis on divine immanence and radical perfectionism. What is interesting is that despite the doctor's theological deviations during the 1890s, SDA leadership failed to act decisively to silence or rebuke him directly in public (Wilson, 2014: 81). A possible explanation, argues Wilson, is that Kellogg's audience was limited primarily to the Battle Creek Sanitarium and a few speaking engagements at conferences, and thus, the stakes were not yet high enough to warrant a public war with America's most famous Adventist (2014: 81). Those sentiments, however, would soon change when *The Living Temple* became public.

In 1903, White wrote personally to Kellogg concerning his views: "You are not definitely clear on the personality of God, which is everything to us as a people. You have virtually destroyed the Lord Himself" (Letter 300, 1903, cited in 5BIO: 292). Within days, White's pen was again active when writing to Kellogg: "Your ideas are so mystical that they are destructive to the real substance, and the minds of some are becoming confused in regard to the foundation of our faith. If you allow your mind to become thus diverted, you will give a wrong mold to the work that has made us what we are — Seventh-day Adventists" (Letter 52, 1903, cited in 5BIO: 292).

Interestingly, White purposed on several occasions at the 1903 General Conference to meet Kellogg's pantheistic teachings face to face in an open meeting exposing the doctor's views in public. Instead, she stated that she was restrained from doing so, and instructed in vision that she "must not say anything that would stir up confusion and strife in the conference" (5BIO: 293). White soon, however, disclosed to President Daniells the underlying forces at play: "Let me tell you . . . Satan has his representatives right here and now at this place, and the Lord has bidden me, have no interview with Dr. Kellogg, no counsel whatever with that man" (5BIO: 241). Interestingly, Douglass insists that the rationale for White's hesitance to confront Kellogg was that the whole controversial episode had to be played out further so that all concerned would see the issues more clearly (1998: 202).

A very brief review of events leading up to the 1903 General Conference is important at this point. On February 1, 1902, the world-renowned Battle Creek Sanitarium was destroyed by fire. Unperturbed, Kellogg within days was requesting financial assistance from the General Conference to rebuild, however, at the time, the denomination was suffering under immense debt. Kellogg was invited to write a popular book on physiology and health care minus any reference to his 'new theories' with the funds received from book purchases going towards the rebuilding of the Sanitarium. Kellogg was impressed and soon began dictating the manuscript for *The Living Temple*. Upon reading the galley proofs, W. W. Prescott and W. A. Spicer were unimpressed, as Kellogg's pantheistic comments were not removed. When news reached Kellogg, he foresaw that the General Conference Committee would withdraw their support and withdrew the manuscript from further consideration as a church sponsored initiative. Kellogg proceeded to place a personal order of 5,000 copies with the Review and Herald Publishing Association, however, on December 30, 1902; a fire reaped the same results with the publishing house as it did ten months earlier with the Battle Creek Sanitarium (Douglass, 1998: 200—203).

Wilson argues that it was Dr. Kellogg's persistent efforts to get *The Living Temple* into publication and available to Adventist readers that brought about White's decision to confront the doctor publically (2014: 87). Thus, when the Autumn Council of the General Conference opened in Washington, D. C., on October 7, the demarcation lines were clearly drawn. After a long day of spirited and heated debate Daniells, the General Conference leader arrived home to be greeted with two messages from Australia bearing White's signature. The messages were unambiguous to say the least:

> I have some things to say to our teachers in reference to the new book The Living Temple. Be careful how you sustain the sentiments of this book regarding the personality of God. As the Lord presents matters to me, these sentiments do not bear the endorsement of God. They are a snare that the enemy has prepared for these last days. . . . It is represented to me that the writer of this book is on a false track. He has lost sight of the distinguishing truths for this time (5BIO: 297, 298).

White metaphorically refereed to the pantheistic issues facing the church as an *iceberg* that must be met head on. "I am instructed to speak plainly," she insisted. "Meet it firmly, and without delay." In Kellogg's book, *The Living Temple* there is "presented the alpha of deadly heresies. The omega will follow, and will be received by those who are not willing to heed the warning God has given" (1SM: 200). With these messages from White now in the public arena and *The Living Temple* available for all to see, the struggles intensified, particularly at Battle Creek.

Was the pantheism crisis in Adventism at the time concerned more with theology or power? Wilson suggests that the two issues were inextricably linked and had much to do with Kellogg's intentions for the future direction of medical missionary work. Wilson's summation is insightful, when stating, "for all his protestations that he honored Seventh-day Adventism's sectarian distinctiveness, it is clear that Kellogg wished to take the denomination in the modernist direction of nondenominational medical ministry work" (2014: 111).

On October 7, 1907, the same year Kellogg was disfellowshipped from the Battle Creek SDA church he was visited by two elders from the church, George Amadon and A. C. Bourdeau, resulting in an interview lasting almost eight hours. Recorded by two of Kellogg's stenographers, the interview fills almost seventy-five pages of single-spaced type. In that interview, Kellogg reiterated that his main goal had been "to make the whole Seventh-day Adventist people a denomination of medical missionaries working . . . to make it the Good Samaritan organization of the world"

(Schwarz, 1990b: 45). To achieve this, declares Wilson, Kellogg was aware that he had to de-emphasize the role of theology in the denomination, and what doctrine there was needed to be elastic enough to accommodate the rapid changes in both science and medicine. Furthermore, this meant forsaking biblical literalism and embracing a theology of immanence more in line with his scientific and medical training. Institutional theology and control, therefore, went together, as perhaps White and other conservative Adventist leaders intuited only too well, and the charges laid against his theology were simply a "convenient but powerful indictment of his modernist agenda for the denomination as a whole" (2014: 111–112). Many individuals who identified with Kellogg's theological position also supported his views regarding control of SDA medical institutions.

Medics, Ministers, and Administrators

By the turn of the twentieth century, Adventism was faced with the need to reorganize due to increased membership and international growth and development. Between 1888 and 1900, a mere twelve years, membership had appreciated by 290 percent, and the movement had a presence in 38 nations. Such rapid growth brought in its wake two significant issues. The first involved financial debt with treasury reports indicating that the church was close to bankruptcy. The year 1900 ended with less than US$50.00 in the treasury, and even that amount was borrowed money (Knight, 2006: 104).

Institutional debt had risen by 1901 to $1.25 million, a very significant amount for that time, and debt was such a burden that the church and its institutions struggled to meet regular interest payments alone. To compound matters further, the General Conference was also responsible for auxiliary organizations even though it exercised minimal control over borrowing processes due to their independent status. This financial burden placed in jeopardy the church's ability to fulfil its obligations to mission outreach through sending missionaries overseas. The President of the Foreign Mission Board reported in 1899 that during the last two years no new work has opened up in any region of the world. It has been an impossibility (*GCDB*, 1899: 73). The second issue facing the church was related to mission. The original, 1863 organizational structures were no longer adequate to service a growing international movement. In other words, the missionary progress and success of the church had begun to demand revisions in the church's administrative structure (Knight, 2006: 105).

Part of the unfinished agenda at the 1901 General Conference involved the incorporation of the medical branch of the Seventh-day Adventist work into the departmental system of the church's organizational structure. The 1901 session had failed to bring the Medical Missionary and Benevolent Association, led by Kellogg into the new unified system, and furthermore, Kellogg wished it to stay that way as he was in no mood for reconciliation. As early as 1890, White had suggested that medical personnel should work under the general direction of local Adventist conferences, an idea that Kellogg had opposed from the start (Schwarz, 2006: 184). "Self-respecting medical men are willing to work on an equal footing with preachers even though they may be of inferior education and ability," Kellogg boldly declared, "but it is not human nature that they could be willing to be slaves to such men while doing their own professional work" (Schwarz, 2006: 184). Kellogg did not believe that the Adventist clergy had any business in a medical institution, and he was as equally determined that none of the medical enterprises he had any association with should ever fall under the control of the Adventist clergy (Schwarz, 2006: 184). Kellogg's views in the early 1900s were somewhat different to those of earlier years for his parents had instilled SDA doctrines into him since early childhood. As an emerging doctor, he expressed his confidence in Adventism declaring, "I sincerely believe the whole truth. I love it and love to work in the cause. I could not be happy anywhere else" (Schwarz, 2006: 178). For over thirty years, Kellogg occupied numerous positions requiring leadership and trust within the SDA movement, all of which ended in 1907 with his official severance of ties with Adventism.

The Clergy—In the Firing Line

Much of the pressure experienced by Adventist leaders around the turn of the twentieth century was caused by the rapid expansion of educational, publishing and medical institutions. Schwarz correctly declares that at an increasing rate, Adventism embodied its message in institutions, for experience had revealed that they were an effective means of evangelism (1986: 123). In addition to constant financial issues, finding appropriate personal to manage the developing institutions was problematic. Furthermore, institutionalization consistently confronted Adventist sectarianism.

Within the education sector, SDA schools were continually admonished to sufficiently differentiate from their secular counterparts to justify their existence. SDA publishing enterprises faced a different set of problems that appeared to have increased in direct proportion to the increase in size of their printing business. Profit margins became the central focus for managers while skilled workers agitated for appropriate remuneration, both of which, argues Schwarz, contributed to the loss of the evangelical zeal that had dictated the founding of an Adventist publishing house in the first place. By 1899 only 40% of the printing completed at the *Review and Herald* was of a religious nature, 20% involved Sanitarium materials, and 40% was strictly secular materials (Schwarz, 1986: 124).

For Kellogg, however, the Adventist clergy were the greatest obstacle in the Seventh-day Adventist cause. Their lackluster approach to health reform promulgated by White and himself remained a constant source of irritation and frustration. Underlying the ongoing power struggle was the conviction by Kellogg and others involved in medical leadership, that the ministerial leadership accepted only a part of the Adventist health message. Some denominational leaders resented Kellogg's enthusiastic endorsement of White's larger view of healthful living, especially in her denunciation of flesh foods, and furthermore, Kellogg found it galling to face criticism of his book, *The Living Temple*, from meat eating denominational leaders (Douglass, 1998: 295).

Kellogg also denigrated the clergy's lack of education in comparison to the medical profession referring to them as men of "very mediocre ability" who maintained their influence and control through "psychological trickery" (Schwarz, 2006: 179). He was particularly skeptical of the minister's lack of financial management and accused them of wasting funds on needless travel, using poor judgement in allocating Adventism's limited finances and for being antagonistic towards medical missionary activities. He also belittled the ministers for being haughty and arrogant.

Clearly, a level of antagonism was reached between Kellogg and the ministry that affected any of the good causes that doctor may have tried to promote. Schwarz summary is compelling when declaring, "unfortunately the doctor never learned the truth of the old saying, 'you catch more flies with honey than with vinegar'" (2006: 179). Again, it would not be overstated to suggest that the clergy's feeling towards Kellogg was, in the main, mutual.

As previously noted, despite Kellogg's incredible success, or perhaps because of it, many members of the Adventist church did not share his zeal for health reform, particularly biological living. Often times, devotees of religious movements, in seeking to maintain doctrinal purity, castigate perceived 'heretics' to the point that any positive contribution made is not acknowledged or simply disregarded. The commonly cited, colloquial term, 'throwing out the baby with the bath water' is a concept used to suggest an avoidable error in which something good is eliminated when trying to get rid of something bad, and perhaps best explains the attitude of many Adventists towards Kellogg. Mistakes were made and words were spoken by real people; various "personalities were involved," and "strongly held convictions were at stake, and human nature was ready," on both sides, "to take pride or offense, as the case may be" (Fiedler, 2014: 120).

Medical institutions imposed their own unique issues, none more as far as Kellogg was concerned, than exposing the lack of technical knowledge and understanding of the clergy in matters of health reform. Kellogg, who had quickly assumed the title of 'czar' over SDA sanitariums, was adamant that he would not take direction from ministerial leaders (Schwarz, 1986: 124). He often complained to White that the majority of SDAs, and particularly the ministers, did not take the health teachings seriously, including White's health reform counsel. The doctor also believed that the clergy were seeking to undermine his influence (Wilson, 2014: 55). Dittes suggests that his correspondence through the years revealed constant challenges as a consequence of opposition from ministers, and in his letters Kellogg would complain of attacks from individuals in the church who he felt should have been his friends (2013: 31).

The Adventist health reform agenda gained momentum following White's Otsego vision in 1865, although it was far from receiving unanimous support by SDAs in practice. Apparently, 'old habits die hard' was an unwritten motto. White, in addition to her constant lecturing, wrote numerous articles concerning health and temperance for various Adventist publications. Adventist temperance efforts reached a crescendo in 1879 with the formation of the American Health and Temperance Association (AHTA) that was presided over by Kellogg. The main agenda of the AHTA was to secure pledges from individuals determining to abstain from tobacco, alcohol, coffee, tea, opium, and all other stimulants and narcotics (Neufeld, 1966: 29–30). White was one of the first to attach her name to teetotal package and one of the most active in signing up others during her constant travels (Numbers, 2008, 229). She was keenly aware of the backsliding and non-adoption of her health reform principles. "Our people are constantly retrograding upon health reform," she stated. "Under the influence of unhealthful food," she continued, "the conscience becomes stupefied, the mind becomes darkened, and its susceptibility to impressions is blunted" (CH: 85).

In 1868, eleven years prior to the establishment of the AHTA, the Seventh-day Adventist Benevolent Association formed to foster support for the many humanitarian needs in society. By 1887, thirty-seven city missions were in operation, however within twelve months; only twenty two were reported, representing a forty percent loss in a single year (*GCDB*: 1888: 26). Three years later, in 1891, Kellogg spoke to the General Conference delegates concerning his research on SDA orphans and the urgent need for his church to be more active in providing funding, resources, and staff to establish an orphanage. Eight days prior to his presentation on the need for an Adventist orphanage at the General Conference session, Kellogg addressed the International Health and Temperance Association, providing his personal perspectives on health reform. The full speech was printed in the *General Conference Daily Bulletin* for all to read. Kellogg, in tandem with White was acutely aware of the retrograde steps being taken concerning health reform practices in Adventism at the time.

An indication of the already deteriorating relationship between Kellogg and the Adventist clergy was clearly evident in his preamble address concerning the Association's activities. The doctor commenced his discussion citing the elevation of health and temperance principles in Adventism, which were adopted by the majority of believers. First alcohol and tobacco were discarded, followed by the consumption of flesh meats in general, and a number of dietary and lifestyle practices were reformed. Unfortunately, by the end of the 1880s, Kellogg insisted, the good work of reform had experienced a marked retrograde to the point that the "promulgation of health principles had ceased to receive the influence necessary to keep them before the people" (*GCDB*, 1891: 41–41). Dr. Kellogg then proceeded to lay the blame for this 'backsliding' progression at the feet of the clergy stating, "no regular means had been provided for systematic consideration of these principles, and as a consequence new converts to the faith received little or no instruction in them." Indeed, significant numbers of young ministers had entered the field as preachers who had never received appropriate instruction in health principles, and as such, "were not prepared either to appreciate their importance or to instruct the people in their precepts" (*GCDB*, 1891: 41–41).

Kellogg was indignant that after many years of counsel from both White and himself the regular use of tea and coffee continued. Even more repugnant was the knowledge that in some instances leading members and officers of the church were found to be habitual consumers of the 'filthy weed'. "There were found among the ministers even, not a few who complained that the pledge was too strong a criticism which from their standpoint was eminently proper, since the pledge evidently prohibited the strong tea to which such critics were almost universally found to be addicted" (*GCDB*, 1891: 41–41).

To add 'insult to injury', Kellogg was particularly agitated at the blatant ignorance towards health reform in evidence when attending Adventist camp meetings. Not only was his presentations timetabled for very early mornings, which irked him considerably, but the camp provision stands prominently displayed all manner of flesh foods including whole codfish, smoked herring, large slabs of halibut, bologna sausage, and dried beef. For years, Numbers argues, Kellogg waged a relentless war; a "one-man crusade" to cleanse the camps of "these odious items" and on occasions, even purchased up the entire stock only to destroy it. He deemed that the "flesh loving campers and ministers constantly hampered his efforts." (2008: 230). At one camp meeting in Indiana, Kellogg paid $15 from his own finances to have the complete stores of meat, strong cheese and some "detestable bakery stuff" deposited in the nearby river, only to discover later that the conference ministers had "surreptitiously salvaged the goods and divided the spoils among themselves" (Numbers, 2008: 230). To Kellogg, the Adventist clergy were the greatest enemies of reform. Many refused to teach and preach against the evils of flesh eating and thus discouraged others who looked to them as examples for guidance (Numbers, 2008: 231). Fiedler insists that while certain aspects of the SDA health reform agenda required a standard of self-denial that not everyone was prepared to adopt, it is another thing to attack the messenger, and there were, unfortunately, some members of the ministry who fell into both of these categories (2014: 123).

White also lamented the fact that the ministry were so belated in adopting reforms that it resulted in Kellogg becoming their harshest critic. "It is a fact that our ministers are very slow to become health reformers, not withstanding all the light which the Lord has given upon the subject," she lamented. Moreover, this has caused Dr. Kellogg to lose confidence in them. "Their tardy work in health reform has created in him a spirit of criticism, and he has borne down on them in an unsparing manner, which the Lord does not sanction," resulting in the denigration of the "gospel ministry," and in his regard and ideas has placed the medical missionary work above the ministry" (4MR: 372).

The disdain Kellogg felt for the clergy filtered through to his relationships with Adventist leaders, and the final decade of his association with the church witnessed particular criticism levelled in that direction. He was indignant that leadership used their influence and bias to lure bright young Adventists into ministry rather than encourage them to enter medical work. The ministry were convinced that Kellogg was pursuing the same aims, only in reverse. Kellogg was further incensed that administration ridiculed his passion for health food creations when first introduced only to become keen to appropriate the profits for use in activities that they controlled when the products became commercially viable (Schwarz, 2006: 178—180).

In a letter to White in 1891, Kellogg wrote of his dismay that some leading men in the church disregarded the work of the Battle Creek Sanitarium as beneficial to the church. "Our doctors have seen that members of the General Conference Committee, and other leading men, did not regard the principles being upheld here, in harmony with the views of the founders of the institution, and the principles laid down in your writings in the Testimonies" Kellogg complained. Furthermore, "they have not attached much importance to these things, and my appeals in the matter have been looked upon as a sort of fanatical zeal" (Kellogg to White, October 2, 1891, Ellen G. White Estate). Kellogg then proceeded to single out a former General Conference President for particular attention. "Eld. Butler pronounced me an extremist before the whole General Conference only three or four years ago; our young doctors heard what he said and knew perfectly well that I had not his support nor the support of others in my work." Kellogg was indignant that this had led others to believe that the so-called principles of the Sanitarium were simply his notions, and of little account, and not principles to be regarded sacredly and earnestly as belonging to the great body of truth. As a consequence of this incorrect method of assessment, Kellogg protested that these same individuals have felt "justified in regarding their relation to the Sanitarium as a mere business one rather than considering it as a great missionary effort in which they were honored in having a part" (Kellogg to White, October 2, 1891, Ellen G. White Estate).

The tensions between Kellogg, church administrators and leaders was further exacerbated by Kellogg's belief that his medical missionary work was disrespected, and held of little value unless it had some pure evangelistic focus resulting in baptized members. (Dittes, 2013: 31). "I have been perplexed to understand some of the teachings of Elder Jones, Prof. Prescott, and Dr. Waggoner" Kellogg remonstrated, for they appear to give the people a basis for such ideas, and particularly the fact that they have shown no interest whatsoever in the Orphan Home work nor any of our benevolent and medical missionary enterprises. For Kellogg, these sentiments provided ample evidence that they "do not consider the sort of work in which I have been engaged, and which has, in fact, occupied my whole life since I was a boy, of any especial value or importance (Kellogg to White, March 21, 1893, Ellen G. White Estate).

By the turn of the twentieth century Kellogg's attitude toward White, her counsel and role became a contentious issue for most SDA leaders, as there was a perception that Kellogg used White's counsel to his own advantage. The doctor held White in high regard and he corresponded extensively with her until his departure from the church. Dittes argues that Kellogg required the ongoing support of the church, which obviously included the endorsement of White to successfully operate his sanitarium and schools in Battle Creek, and that his many personal letters to White appear to be more of an attempt to promote and advance his own programs and agenda (2013: 17). As early as 1899, he complained that there was a conspiracy against him and that someone was misinforming White about his activities. This all served to intensify deteriorating relationships and ensure power struggles for control would continue.

Kellogg had been at odds with virtually every General Conference president since the 1880s, but these tensions were elevated to new heights in the early 1990s when his personal conflict with the incumbent president, Arthur G. Daniells became intense and acidic. Daniells was a competent administrator and one of the very few Adventist leaders that were not intimidated by Kellogg's prowess, and as such, was willing to work with him, at least in public, to promote the medical work of Adventism. Due to increasing financial woes and the enforcement of a no-debt policy by Daniells, which effectively blocked Kellogg's endeavors to establish a sanitarium in England, relationships between the Kellogg and church administration spiraled rapidly downwards. Wilson comments on the impact, declaring that the consequent row, coupled with Daniell's discovery of Kellogg's skepticism of White's prophetic gifts, made Daniells "an implacable foe, more determined than ever to bring the medical work under denominational control" (2014: 109–110). Kellogg's response was to engineer the removal of Daniells from presidency, which failed to materialize. This led to a resolution by Daniells that was approved by General Conference delegate's vote that all Adventist institutions must be owned and administered directly through a General Conference agency. This decision had momentous implications for the future of SDA health institutions, and in response Kellogg retaliated by dissolving the International Medical Missionary and Benevolent Association in 1905, but not before he had transferred its assets to the Battle Creek sanitarium, leaving the General Conference to carry the debts. Wilson argues that these ongoing theological disagreements coupled with tit-for-tat power politics had produced an untenable situation between the denomination's leadership and Kellogg (Wilson, 2014: 110).

Kellogg's anti-clergy agenda and ongoing criticism progressed to matters other than vegetarianism. Adventist ministers, have historically, received special place in the denomination as they are expected, more than all others, "to maintain the ideological and structural foundations" of Seventh-day Adventism (Bull & Lockhart, 2007: 300). White regarded the minister as the rightful advocate of God's truth when declaring that the "minister of Christ has great responsibilities to bear if he would become an example for his people and a correct exponent of his Master's doctrine" (4T: 263). The strategic importance of the minister was a key reason that they quickly assumed dominance within the SDA movement, and adding more weight to their designated position was the acknowledgment by Adventist members that the minister's calling by God was more sacred than any other (Bull & Lockhart, 2007: 300).

Kellogg disputed this rationale and began to illustrate his deep contempt for ministers and their supposed supremacy, running down the ministry in every way possible (Schwarz, 1964: 349). He considered the men who comprised the SDA ministry to be ignorant, uneducated and second-rate individuals and that the standing of a doctor was at least as high as any minister. Formal education for the majority of early Adventists was virtually non-existent. Kellogg, on the other hand, possessed a creative mind that knew no limits. As a physician, cereal maker, inventor, surgeon, educator, administrator, religious leader, public speaker, and author, he crammed the accomplishments of many individuals into one lifetime. With his medical degree, wide reading, extensive travel, both domestic and international, and friends and professional associates from all walks of life, Kellogg lived in a world that most Adventists of the time did not recognize, less understand. His involvement in the health industry brought him to interface with society in numerous ways that consistently challenged Adventism's sectarian positioning in American society. With a reasonable dose of arrogance, Kellogg deemed himself "culturally superior" to the Adventist clergy who possessed "mediocre ability" (Schwarz, 1964: 348–350). He was also very critical of the clergy in their methods of dispensing church funds. "Wasting money" on unnecessary ministerial travel or expenditure on publishing houses, were the words Kellogg used to describe his displeasure. He also frequently lashed out at what he perceived as the dictatorial manner the SDA clergy assumed (Schwarz, 1979: 283).

In view of his attitude, it is not difficult to envisage why Kellogg was so insistent on preventing *any* medical facility, and in particular, the Battle Creek Sanitarium, from coming under the control of the Adventist ministry. Kellogg was further convinced that General Conference leaders were 'bathed with the same brush,' and that they were constantly plotting to gain control of all Adventist institutions. The doctor articulated his underlying grievances on one occasion declaring:

> It seems incomprehensible that men should get so exalted in their own estimation as to form conceptions that a preacher is so much superior to a doctor or a doctor so much inferior to a preacher, that the doctor, or even a company of Christian doctors, would be capable of directing their own work, in which they have been trained for years, while the preacher, who has had no experience in the work whatsoever, becomes by virtue of his ministerial license, competent to direct the physician or the nurse. (Schwarz, 1972: 26, 27)

In visa-versa fashion, throughout this period the Adventist leadership came to fear that Kellogg sought not only to control the church's medical missionary work, but fundamentally change the character of the Seventh-day Adventist movement (Wilson, 2014: 59). It does not require a great leap in one's imagination to understand how this reciprocal ill feeling blossomed to the point that any project or teaching from either party was simply condemned to redundancy.

Ultimately, White sided with the ministry, and perhaps with Kellogg in mind, declared that there must "must be no belittling of the gospel ministry, and furthermore, "no enterprise should be so conducted as to cause the ministry of the word to be looked upon as an inferior matter. It is not so." White stated unequivocally that those who engage in demeaning the Adventist clergy are, in reality, belittling Christ. "The highest of all work is ministry in its various lines, and it should be kept before the youth that there is no work more blessed of God than that of the gospel minister" (6T: 411).

White's unambiguous support for the church's clergy provided a suitable foundation for the professionalization of the Adventist ministry, argue Bull & Lockhart, however, her remarks also brought into sharp focus a deep chasm and conflict between Adventism's ministers and doctors. This conflict was not just about the relative status of these two groups but embodied fundamental differences concerning the identity of Adventism in the future (2007: 301).

In her book, *Medical Ministry*, Ellen White declares the symbiotic relationship that must exist between the medical ministry and gospel ministry arguing that "gospel workers are to minister on the right hand and on the left, doing their work intelligently and solidly," and that there is to exist "*no division between the ministry and the medical work.*" The minister should work equally with the physician, she declared, and with as "much earnestness and thoroughness for the salvation of the soul, as well as for the restoration of the body" (1932: 237, emphasis mine). History records that White's counsel was short lived and that the medical, ministry divorce within Seventh-day Adventism eventuated in the early 1900s. It is to the contemporary implications of that separation that we now turn our attention.

7

Medicalization, Modernization and Change in Adventist Institutionalized Health Care

Impact of Scientific Medicine

IN CHAPTER 2 THE tensions that existed in the nineteenth century between science and religion was discussed, and it was noted that the impact of scientific discovery and method was unprecedented, affecting all strata's of society. No discipline was exempt, including the field of medicine.

Prior to the nineteenth-century America, there were few scientists whose vocation was fully engaged in the pursuit of scientific research (Rogers, 2015: 45). This situation radically changed in the 1800s, however, with the appearance of 'big science,' scientific equipment and the establishment of scientific laboratories for science, Bynum contends, and was one of the most significant factors "in shaping the structure of medicine" in that era. The founding of the Smithsonian Institute in 1846 and the John Hopkins University in 1876 marked the commencement of modern American science (1994, 94–95, 114). Porter concurs arguing that the post-1800 age witnessed the bankrolling of public science, ushering in new institutions, work force, teaching, training and heightened expectations. New scientific bodies were established, the state turned patron and the budding reformers declared "science the dynamo of progress" (1997: 305).

While the impact of science began to slowly permeate all strata's of society, the medically related fields appear to have benefited most from scientific progress. Foucault suggests that medicine made its initial "appearance as a clinical science" in France in 1790 with the establishment of the clinic (cited in Rogers, 2015: 45). Thus, began a permanent relationship between science and physicians upon which, "cutting-edge medicine shifted gradually from the domestic bedside to the hospital and the laboratory" (Numbers, 2011, 206).

The American Civil War (1861–65) also provided another conduit through which the application of science to public health occurred due to the dysentery and typhoid scourges that claimed many lives. Health Boards were established across the nation to regulate standards resulting from ongoing scientific research, which required the training of physicians to staff facilities (Rogers, 2015: 47). Such was need for competent personnel; that estimates suggest that between 1865 and 1915, fifteen thousand American doctors undertook training in German medical centers (Numbers, 2011: 210). The Red Cross was formed in 1863 and the Nursing profession established as a professionally organized occupation during the 1860s and was accompanied during these mid-nineteenth century decades with other specializations including pharmacology, dentistry, antisepsis, anesthetics, obstetrics and surgery (Bynum, 1994: 187–196; Porter, 1997: 375–388).

Another insight into the burgeoning progress in science and medicine involved the development and refining of medical instruments. Technical improvements that reduced distortion brought the microscope from oblivion to the center of biological and medical research. The stethoscope was invented in the nineteenth century as a valuable diagnostic instrument. X-ray technology was discovered in 1895 resulting in their emissions being utilized in the medical field of radiography in 1896 (Rogers, 2015: 45). With the hasty development of printing press networks across the country, the American population was continually informed of these major developments (Bynum, 1994: 173).

By the end of the nineteenth century and resulting from scientific exploration into germ theory, Rogers declares, "the fangs had been drawn from a number of deadly and socially significant diseases" including cholera, tuberculosis, diphtheria, hydrophobia and anthrax (2015: 46). In 1887, the first laboratory for disease diagnosis and monitoring was established in the Staten Island Marine Hospital, which later was transferred to Washington

DC and renamed the Hygienic Laboratory. In quick pursuit, similar projects were launched in Providence and New York.

Thus, by 1900 diagnostic laboratories featured in most major cities in every state and coupled with the integration of science and medical research in the training of physicians in facilities including Harvard, John Hopkins, and the Universities of Michigan and Pennsylvania, it was obvious that modern, scientific based medicine was now embedded in USA society (Porter, 1997: 419–420, 530). Such was the brisk pace of scientific and medical developments that the year 1906 witnessed almost 50% of the world's medical schools located in the USA.

It is of no small significance that J. H. Kellogg graduated from three years medical training at New York's Bellevue Hospital Medical College in 1875 as Adventism's first fully fledged doctor. His life's goal was to continuously broaden the "boundaries of commonly accepted health beliefs and practices," during an era, which not only witnessed rapid advances in medical science, as previously noted, but also an "emerging divide between religion and science" (Skrzypaszek, 2015: 117). The rising profile of scientific and medical achievements continue, to a large degree, to "impress on the public mind the efficacy of science as a provider of solutions to the world's problems," and furthermore, the expansion of scientific technologies during the past century in other areas have confirmed the lifestyle, economic and military benefits "conferred by science." Science, therefore, continues to function, it would appear, as a final court of appeal, that is, "it retains unprecedented authority" despite its status declining somewhat during the past two decades (Rogers, 2015: 62).

The Medicalisation of Adventism (Part 1)

Christian churches in the 2nd century AD faced issues that their founders never encountered including the dual processes of institutionalization and secularization, which have continued throughout history to the present day (Knight, 1995: 23). Ferret, when conducting sociological research into the challenges facing Adventism from its inception argues that the progression from a counter-establishment health reform movement to generally accepted mainstream medical institutions has proved "decisive in providing overall upward mobility for the movement, while simultaneously diluting its sectarianism" (2008: 6). If publishing endeavors instigated the need for SDA organisation, it was the Adventism's foray into medicine that exerted perhaps the most profound impact on the nature of the movement. This process, now known as *medicalization*, deserves further consideration.

The most discernible changes in both public and private behavior globally, has resulted, not only from a decline in religion per se, but rather, to an ever-increasing reliance on governments, corporations and individuals upon the collective knowledge and wisdom of medical and paramedical professionals. The medicalisation process is a universal phenomenon today with people being examined and assessed at every phase in their lifecycle. Physicians, nurses, social workers and psychologists, to name a few, are likely to be consulted at birth, childhood and adolescence. Their assessments are regularly required prior to commencing tertiary studies, employment or initiating life insurance. Their advice is frequently sought regarding conception, gestation and maturation and their opinions are overwhelmingly treated with a respect that verges on reverence—a place in centuries past afforded to the clergy.

It is not just the experience of the individual, however, that is dominated by medical considerations. Food manufacture is monitored by medical experts including commentary on nutritional values. Public health legislation regulates car design while the penalties for deviating from medically sanctioned standards of behavior are severe. Children whose health is impoverished and endangered can be taken from their parents by Government authorities in placed in foster care, immigrants rely on successful medical reports and individuals who fail medical examinations are more likely to experience difficulties in gaining employment and purchasing real estate. People whom a psychiatrist may judge to be far too deviant for the wellbeing of society may be incarcerated, and the list goes on (Bull, 1988: 15–17).

Malcolm Bull argues a strong case when suggesting that modern society continues to be heavily influenced by the process of medicalisation, rather than secularization alone, although the outcome is the same—the elimination of religion from its previously dominant position. It is not that a vacuum now exists; rather, medicine often fulfils the functions previously performed by religion. Bull elaborates further, suggesting that "exorcism is turned into catharsis, the confessional box into the psychiatrist's couch, the index of prohibited books into a list of prohibited substances; sin is reclassified as disease" (1988: 16).

Today, the relative status of medical professionals and the clergy have been reversed, along with the magnitude of their salaries! While one can proceed through life nowadays without the need to contact clergy, the same cannot be said for physicians for even at death a doctor is required to certify termination. The medicalization thesis does not imply that religion is in total retreat per se, rather, "medical practices, and the health related philosophies that legitimate them, have superseded religious values and activities as the predominant guiding force in many areas of social life" (Bull, 1988: 17).

Since the Kellogg era, the process of medicalization provides a core insight and key to understanding many of the significant tensions that exist with Seventh-day Adventism today.

Adventism's expanding medical work has given rise to a "prominence a medical awareness and influence" in the church (Rogers, 2015: 63), so much so argues Bull that medicalization has contributed more to change within Adventism than the more commonly held secularization thesis (1988: 12–21).

Adventist Ministers and Medics—Unequally Yoked?

It was never the intention nor was it anticipated that ministers and physicians would eventually represent alternate interpretations of the Seventh-day Adventist tradition, for both were originally destined like "harnessed horses . . . to pull the Adventist carriage at the same speed, along the same route" (Bull & Lockhart, 2007: 302). Both the medical and clergy personnel were equally as important in spreading the church's message, which was intended to combine a distinctive theology with a unique health reform emphasis. From the mid-1870s, when Kellogg assumed leadership of the Battle Creek Sanitarium in Michigan, changes became evident leading to a redefining of the core of Adventism, including the movement's identity.

The SDA church from its early years has had ministers at the helm. Of the four major nineteenth-century sectarian movements, Adventism was the lone tradition that developed a professional ministry. Neither the Mormons, Jehovah Witnesses or the Christian Scientists did so, nor did they seek to establish theological training schools for without a professional ministry the need for seminaries or their accreditation would have been redundant.

James White, in a series of articles in the *Review* in 1865 viewed the Adventist minister as a type of 'watchman' for the church. This role included the concept of guardianship to warn members of impending dangers, and to prevent sin from entering the church. Ellen White also invoked the metaphor of ministers as watchmen and 'keepers of the gate' as it provided an appropriate framework for her accent on the specific qualities required by the ministers as they protect their flock (4T: 402, 403). She elsewhere described the SDA ministers as "sentinels" who remain always "on duty" and as such, they "are to stand as watchmen on the walls of Zion, to sound the note of alarm at the approach of the enemy" (GW: 15, 451). Thus, the church pastor was responsible for maintaining the ideological and structural foundations of Adventism's alternative society and as such was to be a "correct exponent" of both SDA doctrine and church organizational and institutional endeavors (4T: 263; 1T: 271–272).

Viewed from this perspective, argue Bull and Lockhart, the idea of the ministry as security guards assumes symbolic importance, for Adventist ministers "stand at the gate between the church and an implicitly hostile culture. As such, they maintain a watchful eye on the monster that lurks outside the wall that separates Adventism from the rest of America, and at the first sign of danger, they act as a sort of early warning system for the Adventist community" (2007: 300).

The strategic importance of the ministry provided the mechanism by which they quickly achieved a dominant position within their tradition, however, their ministerial status and supremacy was seriously challenged in the 1890s by Kellogg who became quite vocal in his contempt for Adventist clergy, as previously noted. When speaking of the responsibilities of the physician, White in 1885 penned the following: "Professional men, whatever their calling, need divine wisdom. But the physician is in special need of this wisdom in dealing with all classes of minds and diseases. He occupies a position even more responsible than that of the minister of the gospel" (5T: 439).

Almost simultaneously, White, when seeking to provide mediation through the written page defended the position of the clergy against the continuing verbal barrages of Kellogg, stating that "no enterprise should be so conducted as to cause the ministry of the word to be looked upon as an inferior matter" (6T: 411). White's latter comments brought into sharp focus a deepening conflict between Adventism's clergy and medical professionals. At stake was the nature of SDA identity in the world. Bull and Lockhart's summary is worthy of repetition:

> Insofar as they were called upon to insulate the congregation from a hostile world and to sustain the ideological and structural bases of the church's alternative society, ministers personified the Adventist response to the American nation." On the other hand, Adventist doctors symbolized a new tradition for they were the "first group to mount an effective challenge to the authority of the clergy and to attempt to modify the church's attitude toward the world around it. (2007: 301)

Institutionalization and Secularization

Ellen White's visions and counsel provided the rationale on which the development of Adventist institutions and organizations would be established. It was her central concern that the "establishment of organizations and institutions would prepare people spiritually, physically and mentally for the imminent *parousia*," irrespective of how short or long *imminent* might be interpreted to mean (Ferret, 2008: 304). White was convicted that the motive for establishing institutions was the nearness of the Lord's Advent, rather than a declaration that institution building implied further delay. Her emphasis on institutional evangelism, argues Yamagata, was one of the most distinctive aspects of her understanding of mission (1983: 274).

The rationale for the development of Adventist institutions, according to White was to assist in proclaiming a final warning message to the world, and she was incensed that some of the early Adventist believers were convinced that building institutions was a waste of the Lord's money given the expectant return of the Lord and shortness of time left on earth. Her response was swift to the sentiments from those who insisted that because the Lord is soon to return there is no need to establish schools, sanitariums and food factories. "It is the Lord's design," she argued, "that we shall constantly improve the talents He has given us . . . The prospect of Christ's soon coming should not lead us to idleness. Instead, it should lead us all to do all we possibly can to bless and benefit humanity" (MM: 268).

Seventh-day Adventist institutions were established, therefore, as a 'means to an end.' Institutions were erected to promote, protect and maintain sectarian beliefs and practices in the context of the approaching consummation of the world. The major tension that continues to resonate within the movement, however, is that while Adventist "institutionalism has created space and justification for their separation from secular society; it has also diminished their distinction from the world and questioned the derivation of their identity" (Ferret, 2008: 305). Sociologists note that as institutions grow and interface more with society, there is inevitably an increased need to both recognize and comply with the regulatory requirements of that same society. This inevitable interaction contributes to the ongoing erosion of those distinctive features, which initially characterized and defined the institution, as noted in Chapter 1 (Rogers, 2015: 65).

Adventist education has been the chief factor in lowering Adventism's sectarianism. A core motivation in founding their own educational system was the perceived dread of contamination from outside secular influences and the inevitable erosion of faith as a result. The educative process has become, however, a two-edged sword, in that, while seeking to preserve their sectarian boundaries via these educational institutions, these very same institutions have provided enormous opportunities for member's upward mobility and have generated critical evaluation with many young people opting to pursue other careers, lifestyles and alternative philosophies. The medicalization of Adventism on the basis of its health care system, as has been noted above, has also provided Adventism with its most significant interface with society, however, in the process it has also contributed "further to the movement's respectability, legitimacy and diminishing sectarianism" (Ferret, 2008: 306).

White was patently clear in her assessment as to the intended nature of Adventist institutions when declaring:

> Every institution that bears that name of Seventh-day Adventist is to be to the world as was Joseph in Egypt, and as were Daniel and his fellows in Babylon. In the providence of God these men were taken captive, that they might carry to heathen nations the knowledge of the true God. They were to make no compromise with the idolatrous nations with which they were brought in contact, but were to stand loyal to their faith, bearing as a special honor the name of the worshippers of the God who created the heavens and the earth. (8T: 153)

> As our work has extended and institutions have multiplied, God's purpose in their Establishment remains the same. The conditions of prosperity are unchanged. (6T: 224)

Contemporary SDA Institutionalized Health Care

It is well known that the SDA health message was not original in content, as many health reformers of the era had been advocating similar messages. The health-reform crusades were essentially a lay protest against the orthodox medical practice of the day. The pre-existing health reform package including abstinence from tobacco, alcohol, sex, rich foods and the inclusion of natural remedies was embodied in the thought of Ellen White basically unchanged. An essential difference, however, was that health reform was no longer considered an end in itself, rather, as a means through which the believer could overcome physical cravings that might be satisfied in a sinful way. Health reform, therefore, was religiously motivated and this cut across the grain of existing conventional wisdom. Bull argues that in these important respects, "early Adventist health philosophy differs fundamentally from that of the late 20th century" and it was primarily the work, example and influence of Dr John H. Kellogg that initiated many of these changes (1988: 17).

While scientific research took decades to confirm and endorse SDA beliefs and practices regarding diet and smoking, for example, Dr Kellogg had already prepared the rapprochement between medical orthodoxy and Adventism. The development of the Battle Creek Sanitarium and medical school along with his own personal contacts in the scientific, medical and governmental arenas contributed to aligning Advent medicine in varying degrees with the revitalized medical orthodoxy of the twentieth century.

Kellogg also sought to effect a change in Adventist theology and identity, which along with other factors ultimately led to his demise with Adventism. Bull argues that Kellogg's pantheistic leanings were simply a "spillover for his enthusiasm for health" for he insisted that the spiritual importance of physical health be afforded full recognition (1988: 17). Indeed, Kellogg's passion was to accommodate his biological living themes (also known as the 'Battle Creek Idea') with theological ideals (Wilson, 2014: 175). One example is where Kellogg sought to synthesize physical health with Adventist eschatology. During correspondence with Ellen White in 1898, he challenged Adventism's traditional understanding of the mark of the beast and seal of God, when arguing that obedience to health principles and laws were more important than observance of a particular day of worship. He wrote:

It seems to me our people have been wrong in regarding Sunday observance as the sole Mark of the beast . . . it is simply the change of character and body which comes from the surrender of the will to Satan. (cited in Schwarz, 1972: 24)

During the foundational years of Adventist health care in the late nineteenth century, two types of institutions existed: sanitariums and public clinics. Kellogg's Chicago public clinics were an example. At one time, as many as 12 cities in North America witnessed the presence of Adventist clinics operating on the basis of 'disinterested benevolence' as espoused by White. The purpose of these institutions were to provide medical care for those who were unable to afford it. The pattern of these public clinics were multiplied worldwide and assisted in providing a base for ongoing community service for the church. In countries where these medical ventures proved to be successful, mission hospitals often followed which were funded and supported entirely from church subsidies, with economic gains rarely experienced. Expatriate medical personnel provided the professional services and the mission hospital was intended not only to treat medical conditions, but also to serve an evangelistic function.

Indeed, contemporary Seventh-day Adventism is facing a dynamic reorientation unknown to its pioneers. Science, technology, knowledge, and globalization has developed at a rapid pace. While SDA hospitals in some developing countries continue to adopt a similar medical trajectory as that witnessed in the mid-nineteenth century, the situation is fundamentally different in the majority of other contexts.

In the years since 1907, SDA sanitariums have transitioned to modern medical and surgical institutions, independent of clerical control. Furthermore, both government and medical insurers have increased their respective influence of the broad economics of health care resulting in further erosion of institutional decision-making outcomes. Bevan's analysis is perceptive when declaring that although "few administrators publicly admit the fact, the witness of these institutions involves little direct evangelism and is much like that espoused by James White" (Beaven, 1994, 167).

In the USA and other countries where mission clinics experienced success they often developed into church administered hospitals known as Sanitariums which flourished between 1900 and 1950. These institutions were staffed predominantly by church members and medical staff were primarily local professionals. These institutions were intended to be self-funding with a mandate that employees, including physicians be committed Adventists. Furthermore, physician remuneration was similar to that of SDA clerics.

Between 1950 and 1970 in the USA and some other countries, SDA hospitals changed from church based hospitals to community hospitals. Irrespective of ownership (church or church entity) and while governance links to the church continued, these institutions were no longer operated directly by church administrators, rather, operational administration was provided by professionals. The professionalisation of these hospitals was on the basis that they met or exceeded community quality health care standards. Increasingly, more non—Adventists were employed as medical requirements and treatments advanced, creating friction for many SDA church members who insist that SDA hospitals have aborted their original intention and identity (Beavan, 1994: 165–171).

In his publication "Seventh-day Adventist Health Care—Myth and Reality," Winton Beaven provides valuable insights into the ongoing dilemma. The author declares that the directives provided by Ellen White relate to institutions that no longer exist in most countries. Clinics and sanitariums have been generally replaced by acute care facilities. Adventist medical institutions have been required to change and accommodate advancing technology and delivery of treatment. While Adventists continue to emphasize a wholistic approach to health, incredible changes have occurred in the SDA health care systems, yet Adventist administrators are often reluctant in highlighting those changes. Indeed, as noted previously, many Adventists recognize these changes and vehemently oppose them and have established self-supporting ventures, such as Weimar in the USA. No amount of public relations promotions or praise of Ellen White will "placate those who desire to return to nineteenth-century practices . . . so long as we carry in our minds a false picture of what these institutions were, we are going to have great difficulty in addressing the problems of the present and future" (Beavan, 1994: 168, 169).

A hagiographic picture familiar to many Adventist's is the typical nineteenth century sanitarium description of patients who would visit the dining room where they enjoyed a vegetarian meal, than sat through regular lectures in the parlor that addressed healthful living habits. Tracts were regularly distributed to patients with the intention that these papers might provide an opening to the preaching of the gospel. "This is a lovely picture; I remember it well. I and my family lived with it and enjoyed it." Interestingly, however, the same author states that we cannot draw the conclusion that sanitariums were ever a successful proselytizing agency, instead challenging anyone to provide data that invalidates his view. "If someone is hiding it, it should be brought forward because, unless such data exists, we are carrying a false idea of what our sanitariums accomplished with respect to the mission of the church" (Beavan, 1994: 169). Many rich and famous individuals attended SDA sanitariums, but there is no record that they became Adventist church members as a result, thus, "our picture of SDA sanitariums as being significant soul—winning endeavors is unrealistic. It simply did not happen that way. If it did happen under these ideal conditions, it is entirely unrealistic to expect modern—day hospitals to do any better" (Beavan, 1994: 169, 170).

Of immense significance is that for many Adventists the concept that Adventist sanitariums were able to function effectively and financially as sanitariums that dealt with wholistic health and lifestyle should still be functioning today is somewhat naïve. What appears to be overlooked is the reality that the 'healthstyle' division of SDA hospitals and sanitariums were never an economic success. Beavan argues that they continued because SDA physicians "accepted nominal salaries for their work, thus providing the profits of our sanitariums that enabled them to carry out their healthstyle operation" (1994: 170). There is no indication in SDA history that health-style/healthcare alone has ever been able to support itself economically. "In other words, while we remember the sanitarium, it was the *hospital* end of the institution that enabled it to exist" (Beavan, 1994: 170).

Dave Fiedler, in the book *D'Sozo—Reversing the Worst Evil*, concludes his discussion declaring that on an individual level, Adventist members and ministers must reignite the nineteenth-century blueprint concerning medical/missionary outreach in local communities, originally demonstrated by Jesus and confirmed by Ellen White. Perhaps an equally pressing concern involves the ability for Adventist health institutions to navigate in a world entirely different from that of Christ's and White's era. Fiedler laments the role that the American Medical Association has exerted on the Loma Linda hospital in California, declaring "but did the dragon of Revelation twelve use the AMA to distort our perception of God's call for blended Gospel-Medical Missionary Evangelism? It does seem that way to me." The author while acknowledging the serious challenges facing contemporary SDA health institutions states that "what to do about those challenges, in my ignorance I will keep silent, except to pray for those who are called to face them" (2012: 283, 284). This is no way discredits the author but highlights an ongoing challenge for religious movements birthed in a modernist context seeking to remain relevant in a post-modernist context.

It would appear that the hundreds of pages of instruction provided by White in the nineteenth century concerning SDA sanitariums were time and context specific. While certain principles concerning care are always applicable, specific standards of treatment etc. are not. If Seventh-day Adventism "is to continue as a health care provider, it must make an intelligent adaption of its mission to fit these realities" (Beavan, 1994: 170).

Medicalization of Adventism (Part 2)

Bull (1988: 17) argues that it was undoubtedly the influence Dr. J. H. Kellogg on the basis of his scientific endorsement of Adventist health practices, the establishment of the Battle Creek Sanitarium, the foundation of the medical school and his own personal contacts with the medical and scientific establishments that legitimized much of Adventist health reform, and in the process, edging it closer with "revitalized medical orthodoxy of the early 20th century." While Kellogg was eventually excommunicated from the SDA church, his medical legacy remained. New hospitals were established and a new medical school at Loma Linda was expanded. The net result of this increasing prominence of medicine within Seventh-day Adventism has come closer to realizing the medicalization of Adventism for which Kellogg had wished but never really experienced (Bull, 1988: 17–18).

From an institutional perspective, since the 1920s, SDA medicine remains to this day virtually unencumbered from denominational control, and modern Adventist hospitals exhibit a non-sectarian character, which continues to cause consternation and chagrin for many church administrators and members, as previously noted. The rationale is clear. For Adventist medicine to survive and exist profitably in the twenty-first century and beyond it has been forced to "follow the lead set by medical orthodoxy, either through the need for accreditation, or else under the force of economic pressure created by heavy competition" (Bull, 1988, 18).

It often goes unnoticed or taken for granted that there should be a state or government monopoly over medical care services, and that unregistered or unqualified practitioners should be differentiated. In significant contrast, the prospect of a government enforced religious monopoly is Adventism's eschatological nightmare. It is also of interest that the General Conference of SDA has a religious liberty department devoted to the maintaining of a free market in religion, which creates some ambiguity. While the religious activities of Adventism worldwide take place in an un-regulated open market, its medical institutions and mission, ('right arm of the gospel') functions as a licensed, registered and constituent part of governmental legislation. Bull declares, "the discrepancy in the operating environments of the two major forms of the Adventist work has been of the most significance" (1988: 18).

SDA's medical endeavors are regulated and limited due to reliance on government policy, while the rest of the church, thus far, exists in an almost unregulated religious market. "Through its simultaneous aversion to religious monopoly, and acceptance to medical monopoly, Adventism ensures wrenching conflicts within the church" (Bull, 1988: 18). There are many more academic discussions concerning Adventist theology than there is regarding medical institutions, and there are calls for democracy at the General Conference but very few for democracy in Adventist hospitals. Ferret argues that in terms of identity, what "SDAs incarnate is *equally* important as what they articulate" (2008: 307).

It would appear that the SDA health-care system, including institutions is in important ways much closer to the Kellogg model than to Ellen White's for the "system has long since abandoned features of White's program, including ministerial pay for physicians, drugless therapy, sexual segregation in doctor/patient relations and many others." Furthermore, "Adventist hospitals are confederated in businesslike organizations that dwarf the General Conference. They do, however, meet the goals of James White" (Beavan, 1994: 168).

There is little doubt that Kellogg was interested in mission. Indeed, every student admitted to his medical school was required to sign a pledge indicating their dedication to a life of medical missionary work. However, as Knight argues, Kellogg's pursuits "brought him face to face with the Adventist dilemma between immediacy and occupancy in a way that other Adventist leaders never had to deal with. Adventist ministry, for example, was "insulated from the direct effect of a secular culture and acceptance by that culture." In contrast, Kellogg's endeavors "took place on the boundary between the larger culture and the church." Thus, in order to successfully engage with 'outsiders, 'Kellogg "had found it profitable to mute his Adventism" (1995: 154, 155).

Many Seventh-day Adventists continue to navigate the dilemma in seeking to "turn back the clock" to the nineteenth century. In the Western world current conditions effectively render impotent the "carrying out in any detail some significant parts of the perceived mission of the church with respect to health care," and as such "if the church is to continue as a health-care provider, it must make an intelligent adaptation of its mission to fit these realities" (Beaven, 1994: 170). The same author concludes by suggesting that a radical change in thought and processing will be required by church members who believe that the directives provided by White for the operation of Adventist sanitariums were both unnegotiable and for all time (1994: 170, 171).

Thus, Seventh-day Adventists continue to struggle with the dual challenges of continuity and change. Perceptions of change never remain static, however, but alter with time. This close connection between identity and time can exert a corrosive effect on identity, particularly for movements, which preach and teach an imminent advent. Knight underscores three methods of relating to change that have confronted many Christian bodies. One is to exist in the past as if the past can be perpetually reserved intact as a golden era. A second dysfunctional method of relating to history and change is to focus exclusively on the future, whilst a third way of relating to change is to forget the future and past and focus exclusively on the present. Knight suggests a fourth method that is anchored in both God's leading both in the past, present and future. "Thus it sets forth a present orientation in the framework of the continuum of the past and the future" (1995: 158).

Adventism continues its journey as it seeks to fulfil its destiny and commission as a pilgrim people, guided by the past, yet simultaneously, continually pressing towards their eventual goal. C. E. Bradford (1979: 6) eloquently stated the challenge:

> A movement is not a settlement; a movement is not a theological point of view. A movement, in the strictest sense, is not a denomination. A movement is a pilgrimage, a people on a journey, an expedition.

Bibliography

Anderson, E. (2014). "War, Slavery, and Race." In T. Dopp Aamodt, T., G. Land & R. L. Numbers (Eds.), (2014). *Ellen Harmon White: American Prophet* (262–278). New York: Oxford University Press.

Ball, B. (1981). *The English Connection.* Cambridge: James Clarke.

Beaven, W. H. (1994). "Seventh-day Adventist Health Care—Myth and Reality." In S. Proctor, E. Durand & R. Gainer (Eds.). *Health 2000 and Beyond: A Study Conference of Adventist Theology, Philosophy, and Practice of Health and Healing.* Wahroonga, NSW: Adventist health Department, South Pacific Division of SDA.

Blake, J. B. (1974). *Health Reform*, in *The Rise of Adventism*, Gaustad, E. S. (Ed.). New York: Harper & Row.

Buettner, D. (2005). "The Secrets of Long Life." *National Geographic.* http://ngm.nationalgeographic.com/ngm/0511/feature1/.

Bull, M (1988). "The Medicalization of Adventism." *Spectrum*, 18:3: 12–21.

Bull, M., & Lockhart, K. (2007). *Seeking a Sanctuary: Seventh-day Adventism and the American Dream.* (2nd ed.). Bloomington: Indiana University Press.

Burt, M. D. (2002). *The Historical Background, Interconnected Development, And Integration of the Doctrines of the Sanctuary, The Sabbath, and Ellen G. White's Role in Sabbatarian Adventists from 1844 to 1849.* Ph.D. diss., Andrews University, MI.

Butler, J. M. (1970). "Ellen G. White and the Chicago Mission." *Spectrum*, 2 (Winter): 41-51.

———— (2014). A Portrait. In T. Dopp Aamodt, T., G. Land & R. L. Numbers (Eds.), (2014). *Ellen Harmon White: American Prophet* (1 – 29). New York: Oxford University Press.

———— (2014). Second Coming. In T. Dopp Aamodt, T., G. Land & R. L. Numbers (Eds.), (2014). *Ellen Harmon White: American Prophet* (178–195). New York: Oxford University Press.

Campbell, M. W. (2008). *The 1919 Bible Conference and Its Significance for Seventh-day Adventist History and Theology.* Ph.D. diss., Andrews University, Berrien Springs, MI.

Carter, P. A. (1971). *The Spiritual Crisis of the Gilded Age.* DeKalb: Northern Illinois University Press.

Coon, R. (1993). "The Good Old Days." *Adventist Review,* 25 February.

Craig, W. J. (1991). "In the Pink of Health." *Adventist Review,* Vol 14, No. 2, Fall Issue.

Crow, K.E. (1993). "The Church of the Nazarene and O'Dea's Dilemma of Mixed Motivation." http://www.nazarene.org/cg/research/ansr /articles/t17.html.

Damsteegt, P. G. (1977). *Foundations of the Seventh-Day Adventist Message and Mission.* Grand Rapids: Eerdmans.

———, (1978). "Health Reform and the Bible in Early Sabbatarian Adventism." *Adventist Heritage* 5, No. 2: 13–21.

Dick, E. N. (1986). "The Millerite Movement, 1830–1845. In G. Land (Ed.). *Adventism in America.* (1–36). Grand Rapids: Eerdmans.

Dittes, A. (2013). *Three Adventist Titans: The Significance of Heeding or Rejecting the Counsel of Ellen White.* Ringgold, GA: Teach Services, Inc.

Doan, R. A. (1987). *The Miller Heresy, Millennialism, and American Culture.* Philadelphia: Temple University Press.

Dopp Aamodt, T., Land, G., & Numbers, R. L. (Eds.). (2014). *Ellen Harmon White: American Prophet.* New York: Oxford University Press.

———. (2014). Speaker. In T. Dopp Aamodt, T., G. Land & R. L. Numbers (Eds.). *Ellen Harmon White: American Prophet* (110–125). New York: Oxford University Press.

Douglass, H. E. (1998). *Messenger of the Lord: The Prophetic Ministry of Ellen G. White.* Nampa, ID: Pacific.

Eiseley, L. (1970). *The Invisible Pyramid.* New York: Scribner.

Engs, R. C. (2000). *Clean Living Movements: American Cycles of Health Reform.* Westport,

Fielder, D. (2102). *D'SOZO: Reversing the Worst Evil.* Coldwater, MI: Remnant.

Gaustad, E. S. (Ed.). (1974). *The Rise of Adventism.* New York: Harper & Row.

Gaustad, E., & Schmidt, L. (2002). *The Religious History of America.* San Francisco: HarperCollins.

Graybill, R. (2014). Prophet. In T. Dopp Aamodt, T., G. Land & R. L. Numbers (Eds.), (2014). *Ellen Harmon White: American Prophet* (74–90). New York: Oxford University Press.

Greenleaf, F., & Moon. J. (2104). Builder. In T. Dopp Aamodt, T., G. Land & R. L. Numbers Oxford University Press.

Haller, J. S. Jr. (1981). *American Medicine in Transition, 1840–1910.* Urbana: University of Illinois Press.

Hancock, T. (1992). The Healthy City: Utopias and Realities. In J. Ashton, J (Ed.). *Healthy Cities.* Milton Keynes, UK: Open University Press.

Hanks-Harwood, G. (1995). Wholeness. In C. W. Teel, Jr. (Ed.). *Remnant and Republic: Adventist Themes for Personal and Social Ethics.* Loma Linda, CA: Center for Christian Bioethics.

Hardinge, M. G. (2001). *Drugs, Herbs & natural Remedies.* Hagerstown, MD: Review & Herald.

Heyrman, C. L. (2000). "The First Great Awakening." (online). http:www.nhc.rtp.nc.us/ Serve/eighteen/ekeyinfo/grawaken.html.

Hudson, W. S. (1974). "A Time of Religious Ferment." In R. G. Gaustad (Ed.). *The Rise of Adventism* (1–17). New York: Harper and Row.

Jackson, W. (2015). "The Nineteenth-Century Context of the Seventh-day Adventist Health Message." In. L. J. Rogers (Ed.). *Changing Attitudes to Science within Adventist Health and Medicine from 1865 to 2015*. Cooranbong, NSW: Avondale Academic.

Kellogg, J. H. (1879). *Health Reformer*, vol. 14, January.

———. (1879). *Harmony of Science and the Bible on the Nature of the Soul and the Doctrine of the Resurrection*. Battle Creek, MI: Review & Herald.

———. (1886). Letter to E. G. White from Battle Creek, MI, dated June 12, 1886.

———. (1890). *Preface* to *Christian Temperance and Bible Hygiene*. E. G. White. Mountain View, CA: Pacific.

———. (1893). *The Household Monitor of Health*. Battle Creek, MI: Good Health.

———. (1897). [1] *Health and Spirituality*, General Conference Daily Bulletin, Lincoln, Nebraska, 24 February, Vol.1, No. 9.

———. (1897). [2] *God in Nature*, General Conference Daily Bulletin, Lincoln, Nebraska, 18 February, Vol. 1, No. 5.

———. (1897). [3] *Christian Help Work*, General Conference Daily Bulletin, Lincoln, Nebraska, 8 March, Vol. 1, No. 17.

———. (1897). [4] *God in Man*, General Conference Daily Bulletin, Lincoln, Nebraska, 22 February, Vol 1. No. 7.

———. (1898). *City Medical Missions*. Battle Creek, MI: Kellogg Papers.

———. (1898). *Medical Missionary*. January.

———. (1899). *Medical Missionary*. May.

———. (1902). *Ladies Guide in Health and Disease*. Battle Creek. MI: Modern Medicine.

———. (1903). *The Living Temple*. Battle Creek, MI: Good Health.

———. (1904). *The Miracle of Life*. Battle Creek, MI: Good Health.

———. (1905). *Medical Missionary*, XIV, March.

———. (1906). "True Christianity a Medical Missionary Movement," *Medical Missionary* 15, No. 5: 129–133)

———. (1908). "The Degeneration of the Negro." Battle Creek, MI: *Good Health*.

———. (1910). *Life, Its Mysteries and Miracles: A Manual of Health Principles*. Battle Creek: MI: Modern Medicine.

———. (1913). *The Battle Creek Sanitarium System*. Battle Creek, MI: n.p.

———. (1916). *Ideas*. Battle Creek, MI: Good Health.

———. (1921). *The New Dietetics*. Battle Creek, MI: Modern Medicine.

———. (1932). *How to Have Good Health through Biological Living*. Battle Creek, MI: Modern Medicine.

———. (1938). Script of a talk given at Battle Creek Sanitarium, dated 21 October.

Knight, G. (1993). *Millennial Fever and the End of the World*. Boise, ID: Pacific.

———, (1995). *The Fat Lady and the Kingdom*. Boise, ID: Pacific Press Publishing Association.

———. (1998). *Ellen White's World*. Hagerstown, MD: Review and Herald.

———. (1998). *A Friendly Guide to the 1888 Message*. Hagerstown, MD: Review & Herald.

———. (2001). *Organizing to Beat the Devil: The Development of Adventist Church Structure*. Hagerstown, MD: Review & Herald.

———. (2006). *Organizing for Mission and Growth: The Development of Adventist Church Structure*. Hagerstown, MD: Review & Herald.

———. (2007). *If I Were the Devil: Contemporary Challenges Facing Adventism.* Hagerstown, MD: Review & Herald.

Land, G. (1986). *Adventism in America.* Grand Rapids: Eerdmans.

Mann, H. (1868). "The Study of Physiology in the Schools," Educational Annual Report for 1842, *Annual Reports on Education,* (ed.). Mary Tyler Mann, vol. 3. *Life and Works of Horace Mann.* Boston: Horace B. Fuller.

Martin, E. G. (1942). *The Standard of Living in 1860.* Chicago: Ill: University of Chicago Press.

Marsden, G. M. (1982). *Fundamentalism and American Culture.* New York: Oxford University Press.

Mayfield, J. (1982). *The New Nation: 1800–1845.* New York: Hill & Wang.

McGraw, P., & Valentine, G. (2014). "Legacy." In T. Dopp Aamodt, T., G. Land & R. L. Numbers (Eds.). *Ellen Harmon White: American Prophet* (305 – 321). New York: Oxford University Press.

McLoughlin, W. G. (1974). "Revivalism." In E. G. Gaustad, (Ed.). *The Rise of Adventism.* (119–153). New York: Harper and Row.

McMahon, D. S. (2005). *Acquired or Inspired? Exploring the Origins of the AdventistLifestyle.* Victoria, Australia: Signs.

Morgan, D. (2001). *Adventism and the American Republic.* Knoxville, TN: The University of Tennessee Press.

———. (2014). "Society." In T. Dopp Aamodt, G. Land & R. L. Numbers (Eds.), *Ellen Harmon White: American Prophet* (224 – 243). New York: Oxford University Press.

Neufeld, D. F. (1966). (Ed.). "American Temperance Society." *Seventh-day Adventist Encyclopedia.* Washington, D.C.: Review and Herald.

Niebuhr, H. R. (1937). *The Kingdom of God in America.* Chicago: Willet, Clark.

Nieman, D. C. (1992). *The Adventist Healthstyle.* Hagerstown, MD: Review and Herald.

Numbers, R. L. (2008). *Prophetess of Health: Ellen G. White and the Origins of Seventh-day Adventist Health Reform.* (3rd ed.). Grand Rapids: Eerdmans.

Numbers, R. L., & Schoepflin, R. B. (2014). "Science and Medicine." In T. Dopp Aamodt, T., G. Land & R. L. Numbers (Eds.), *Ellen Harmon White: American Prophet* (196–223). New York: Oxford University Press.

Patrick, A. (2014). "Author." In T. Dopp Aamodt, T., G. Land & R. L. Numbers (Eds.), *Ellen Harmon White: American Prophet* (91 – 109). New York: Oxford University Press.

Paulson, D. (1916). Letter in *Paulson Articles and Misc.* Ellen G. White Estate Document File 269a.

Plantak, Z. (1998). *The Silent Church: Human Rights and Adventist Social Ethics.* London: Macmillan.

Proctor, S. & L. (1991). "Searching for the Fountain of Youth." Hagerstown, MD: The Health Connection.

Reid, G. W. (1982). *A Sound of Trumpets,* Washington, DC: Review & Herald.

———. (1994). "Out of Darkness, Light: Roots of Adventist Health Reform." In G. Swanson & E. Durand (Eds.), *Health 2000 and Beyond: A Study Conference of Adventist Theology, Philosophy, and Practice of Health and Healing.* Sydney, Australia: Adventist Health Department, South Pacific Division of SDA.

Robinson, D. E. (1965). *The Story of Our Health Message.* 3rd. ed. Nashville: Southern.

Rock, C. B. (1988). "Did Ellen White Downplay Social Work?" *Advent Review,* 5 May.

Rogers, L. J. (2015). "Science: Once Rejected by the Prophet but Now Profiting Adventist Health." In. L. J. Rogers (Ed.). *Changing Attitudes to Science within Adventist Health and Medicine from 1865 to 2015.* Cooranbong, NSW: Avondale Academic.

Rowe, D. L. (2008). *God's Strange Work: William Miller and the End of the World.* Grand Rapids: Eerdmans.

Schaefer, R. A. (1977). *Legacy.* Mountain View, CA: Pacific.

Scharnborst, G. (1994). "1844 in Great American Literature." *Spectrum,* 24 (2): 28–41.

Schoepflin, R. B. (1987). "Health and Health Care." In G. Land (Ed.), *The World of Ellen White.* Washington, D. C.: Review and Herald.

Schwarz, R. W. (1964). *John Harvey Kellogg, M.D.* PhD diss., University of Michigan.

———. (1969). "John Harvey Kellogg: Adventism's Social Gospel Advocate." *Spectrum,* 1 (Spring): 15–28.

———. (1972). "The Kellogg Schism: The Hidden Issues." *Spectrum,* 4 (Autumn): 23–29.

———. (1979). *Light Bearers to the Remnant.* Boise, ID: Review & Herald.

———. (1986). "The Perils of Growth." In G. Land (Ed.). *Adventism in America.* (95-138). Grand Rapids: Eerdmans.

———. (1990a). "Kellogg vs. The Brethren: His Last Interview as an Adventist—October 7, 1907." *Spectrum, 20*(3), 46–62.

———. (1990b). "Kellogg Snaps, Crackles, and Pops: His Last Interview as an Adventist—Part 2." *Spectrum, 20*(4), 37–61.

———. (2006). *John Harvey Kellogg: Pioneering Health Reformer.* Hagerstown, MD: Review & Herald.

Schaefer, R. A. (2005). *Legacy Daring to Care: The heritage of Loma Linda University Medical Center.* Loma Linda, CA: Legacy.

Schwarz, R. W., & Greenleaf, F. (1995). *Light Bearers: A History of the Seventh-day Adventist Church.* Nampa, ID: Pacific.

Selye, H. (1974). *Stress Without Distress.* New York: A Signet Book.

Seventh-day Adventist Bible Commentary. F. D. Nichol (Ed.). (7 Vols.). 1957; rev. d. 1976-1980). Washington, DC: Review & Herald.

Shi, D. E. (2001). *The Simple Life: Plain Living and High Thinking in American Culture.* Athens: University of Georgia Press.

Skrzypaszek, J. (2015). "John Harvey Kellogg: A case Study of Transforming Health Science." In. L. J. Rogers (Ed.). *Changing Attitudes to Science within Adventist Health and Medicine from 1865 to 2015.* Cooranbong, NSW: Avondale Academic.

Smith, T. L. (1974). "Social Reform: Some Reflections on Causation and Consequences." In R. G. Gaustad (Ed.). *The Rise of Adventism.* (18–29). New York: Harper & Row.

Spalding, A. W. (1962). *Origin and History of Seventh-day Adventists* (4 vols.). Washington, DC: Review & Herald.

Taves, A. (1999). *Fits, Trances, and Visions: Experiencing Religion and Explaining Experience from Wesley to James.* Princeton: Princeton University Press.

———. (2014). Visions. In T. Dopp Aamodt, T., G. Land & R. L. Numbers (Eds.), *Ellen Harmon White: American Prophet* (30–51). New York: Oxford University Press.

Theobald, R. (1979). *The Seventh-day Adventist Movement: A Sociological Study with Particular Reference to Great Britain.* Ph.D. diss. supplied by The British Library Document Supply Centre.

Wacker, G. (2014). Foreword. In T. Dopp Aamodt, T., G. Land & R. L. Numbers (Eds.), (2014). *Ellen Harmon White: American Prophet* (ix–xiv). New York: Oxford University Press.

Walls, A. (1990). The American Dimension in the History of the Missionary Movement. In Carpenter, J. A., & Shenk, W. R. (Eds.). Grand Rapids: Eerdmans.

Weigold, I. B. (2007). *Hannah Moore: A Biography of a Nineteenth Century Missionary and Teacher.* Bloomington, IN: iUniverse.

Wentz, R. E. (2003). *American Religious Traditions.* Minneapolis: Fortress.

Werbach, M. R. (1986). *Third Line Medicine.* New York: Arkana.

Willis, R. J. B. (2003). *The Kellogg Imperative: John Harvey Kellogg's Unique Contribution To Healthful Living.* Grantham, UK: Stanborough.

White, A. L. (1981–1986). *Ellen G. White.* (6 Vols.). Washington, DC: Review and Herald.

White, E. G. (1911). *The Acts of the Apostles.* Mountain View, CA: Pacific.

———. (1923). *Fundamentals of Christian Education.* Nashville: Southern.

———. (1923). *Testimonies to Ministers.* Nashville: Southern.

———. (1923). *Counsels on Health.* Nashville: Southern.

———. (1932) *Medical Ministry.* Mountain View, CA: Pacific.

———. (1938). *Counsels on Diet and Foods.* Washington, DC: Review & Herald.

———. (1940). *The Desire of Ages.* Mountain View, CA: Pacific.

———. (1943). *Life Sketches of Ellen White.* Mountain View, CA: Pacific Press.

———. (1943). *The Story of Prophets and Kings.* Mountain View, CA: Pacific.

———. (1945). *Spiritual Gifts.* (4 Vols.). Washington, DC: Review & Herald.

———. (1945). *Early Writings.* Washington, DC: Review & Herald.

———. (1946). *Christ's Object Lessons.* Washington, DC: Review & Herald.

———. (1946). *Evangelism.* Washington, DC: Review & Herald.

———. (1948). *Testimonies to the Church.* (9 Vols.). Mountain View, CA: Pacific.

———. (1950). *The Great Controversy between Christ and Satan: The Conflict of the Ages in the Christian Dispensation.* Mountain View, CA: Pacific.

———. (1951). *Counsels on Health.* Mountain View, CA: Pacific.

———, (1952). *Education.* Mountain View, CA: Pacific.

———, (1958). *Selected Messages from the Writings of Ellen G. White,* (3 vols.). Washington, DC: Review & Herald.

———, (1958). *The Story of Patriarchs and Prophets.* Mountain View, CA: Pacific.

———. (1961). *Our High Calling.* Washington, DC: Review & Herald.

———. (1962). *Testimonies to Ministers and Gospel Workers.* Mountain View, CA: Pacific.

———. (1981). *Manuscript Releases.* (Vol. 1.) Washington, DC: Ellen G. White Estate.

White, J. B. (1993). *Taking the Bible Seriously.* Louisville: Westminster/John Knox.

Whorton, J. (1982). *Crusaders for Fitness.* Princeton: Princeton University Press.

Wilson, B. C. (2014). *Dr. John Harvey Kellogg and the Religion of Biological Living.* Bloomington: Indiana University Press.

Wolfgramm, R. (1983). *Charismatic Deligitimation in a Sect: Ellen White and Her Critics.* M.A. thesis, Chisholm Institute of Technology, Canberra, Australia.

Milton Keynes UK
Ingram Content Group UK Ltd.
UKHW022156091123
432302UK00005B/44